# Black Market Medicine

"A thought-provoking, taut, and suspenseful read... Through the experience of diverse characters, Cassandra Collins will make you consider and possibly rethink your position concerning the present and future of medical care in America."

Judy-Lynn Goldenberg, Retired Attorney at Law and Senior Lecturer, Johns Hopkins University.

# Black Market Medicine

A NOVEL BY

## Cassandra Collins

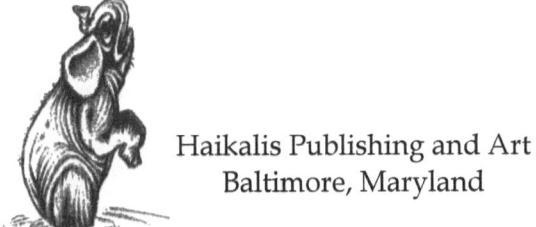

Haikalis Publishing and Art
Baltimore, Maryland

ISBN 978-0-615-41809-4
Library of Congress Control Number 2011913374

Editing and type design: Tracy Collins
Graphic design for cover: Elizabeth Collins
Cover art: Peter Collins
Website and blogmaster: David Collins
Technical advisor: Keri Collins

Printed in the United States of America.

For David...

And for "dinosaurs" like him
—the few physicians still caring for
patients in solo private practices—
who mourn the loss of medical
knowledge and the art of
physical diagnosis.

And for my grandfather,
George Nickolaus…

Who lost a thriving business when
he followed the laws of prohibition,
refusing to sell alcoholic beverages.

For six months in 1933, he visited
a church every morning before
spending the day looking for work,
which he finally found as a waiter.

# U.S. Healthcare Distribution System Act of 2045

1. The United States Federal Government will be the sole provider of all healthcare for its citizens.

2. All United States Citizens are members of The United States Medical Grant of Care Health Delivery System.

3. Citizens may register complaints regarding their healthcare only with the Judicial Branch of the Medical Grant of Care Health Department. Citizens will be permitted to file complaints only one time per health issue. No appeals will be granted, and no other course of action will be tolerated.

4. Prospective doctors, nurses, technicians, and ancillary personnel must pass an aptitude test before being allowed to proceed with training in their respective fields of interest.

5. Each year a nonpartisan board under the auspices of the U.S. Healthcare Distribution System Act will release a list of allowable treatments, therapies, and medicines. The System Board may alter these lists at any time. Notice to citizens in advance is not required.

6. All treatment for any health issue must follow the guidelines provided in the U.S. Healthcare Distribution System Act of 2045 Caregiver Guidelines for Care. Caregivers are expected to stay current with these guidelines as they are reviewed regularly and amended as is deemed appropriate by the U.S. Healthcare Distribution System. Failure to follow these guidelines will result in seizure of license to deliver care as well as consideration of criminal prosecution.

7. All medical research proposals will be reviewed for approval by the U.S. Healthcare Distribution System Board. This will include but is not limited to: all curative techniques, treatment plans, surgeries, medicines, and prosthetic devices.

8. All medical information will be stored on a dedicated computer system to be accessed only by approved personnel.

9. Any citizen involved in treatment or diagnosis outside this plan whether as caregiver or patient will be prosecuted to the fullest extent of the law.

10. Medical Care activities may not be carried out anywhere other than in an approved government structure.

# PROLOGUE

Year 2075

The man on the street had said Condo 420 on Paca Street. She found it easily. She shifted the baby she held to her left arm and knocked on the grimy door, gently at first. Even though it was winter and the heat wasn't on in the hallway, Sharon felt herself sweat. To go underground like this. Never would she have imagined herself capable. Her friends would be amazed. What if she ended up in jail? Who would care for Lily? She looked down at Lily's beautiful face. Pale, very pale, but beautiful. She pulled her closer to her chest and breathed deeply. She had to do this. Lily had to live.

She knocked again on the door. Harder this time. This had to be the place. Her baby had to have care. Finally, the door opened. The man, who had opened the door, small in stature, older than she would have thought, grunted at her to enter. The room was crowded but eerily quiet. Humanity of all sorts filled the room. Eyes all downcast. Some seated on tired sofas, others on the mismatched chairs shoved into any space they would fit. Children as well as adults sleeping on the floor using jackets as pillows. Then there was the smell. That sick hospital smell coupled with the odor of unwashed, damp bodies. Sharon stepped inside and looked around hoping for a friendly look, encouragement from any quarter. She found none. The tension of fear filled the room. Desperation and fear. She didn't want to be here. This was the lowest and last stop on the failed healthcare system in America. There was a day when she never knew of this place. A day when she never knew fear. But here she was. Her pure, angelic baby had brought her to this place of fear and hopelessness. The strange old man had disappeared, without a word, through the door in the back corner of the room. She timidly walked to the opposite corner where there was a small space against the wall. She eased down to her knees careful not to disturb Lily and then sat with her back to the wall. There, she waited.

Hours had passed; she couldn't say how long. She lay on the floor with Lily lying between her and the wall, so no one would inadvertently step on her. Someone was touching her shoulder pulling her out of her semi-sleep state. A woman this time.

"It's time," she said. "Follow me." Sharon quickly gathered her belongings and gently lifted Lily, who stirred, startled by the motion. A small sound came from her mouth to protest being awakened, but she settled back against her mother's breast and resumed sleep.

As they passed through the door, the woman turned to her and said simply, "The money?" Sharon quickly nodded and reached into her pocket to pull out the envelope of money she had been instructed to bring. The woman took it and indicated to Sharon that she was pleased by its contents. They traveled down a narrow hall to a small examining room which the nurse, or whatever she was, nodded for her to enter. Sharon looked around the room hopefully. Her hopes were not answered. The room was dirty. The floor filthy with the dirt tracked by many before her. No diplomas hung on the wall. Only a table and two chairs filled the tiny room. She noticed the absence of a sink. She could leave even now. But then what? This was her last stop. Lily's last stop. This had to work. It had to be the answer. There were no others.

With no warning, the door flew open and a doctor(?) entered swiftly.

"What's her diagnosis," he demanded. She told him.

"Let me have her," he said gruffly and a bit tiredly. The mother naturally resisted.

"I have others waiting. Do you want me to fix this or not?"

She quietly handed Lily to the doctor or whoever he was. He none too gently put Lily on the table and hooked her up to a computer. Lily roused a bit and complained a bit with a whine. The doctor worked quickly, efficiently and without any empathy that the mother could see. Lily might as well have been just another computer.

He looked up. "Do you have her records?" She silently handed them over. He glanced over them quickly. "I agree with this diagnosis. Do you want me to treat her?"

"Of course."

"It will cost more. Operations cost more. They should have told you."

"They did. I'll get whatever you need."

"OK. You can leave her and go now. Come back tomorrow afternoon around four. Bring more money. Talk to no one of this. We're taking a big chance here for you. Keep that in mind." He had already dismissed her.

"But can't I stay?"

"Nope. You can't. Do you want me to treat her or not? I've got other patients to see."

"Yes, do you think you can cure her?"

"Should work OK." He quickly disconnected Lily from the computer, picked her and her medical records up, and left the room.

# CHAPTER 1

Now she knew there was no God. Janis had long been a believer, but no more. Her body had failed her, and so had her God. For three days, she had asked God to take her from this life. Three long torturous days filled only with the hell of pain so intense she felt at times she must be losing consciousness. The cancer had spread. There was no hope and not the slightest given from Caregiver No. 42.

A glass of water, a wet rag on her forehead, even some word of prayer would have been something. She knew they had cut back her allotment of medicine. She had heard that, as late as 2018, there had still been some Wellness Spas that had provided spiritual assistance. Naturally, Janis knew she shouldn't even be thinking such foolish thoughts, but her mother had laid the seed of spiritualism in her many years before. Before the legislation of 2045.

In her assigned Wellness Spa bed she suffered in silence, unable to reach anyone for what seemed like days. Time had lost meaning. The pain kept her from moving. If she lay still, she could just barely tolerate the agony. She decided to reach for the call button sitting tantalizingly close on the bed rail to her left. Movement would hurt, she knew, but she needed something, anything. Cautiously, lest she set off her pain, she slid her arm to the left, eyes on the red button. She had accomplished this once before, and she knew her index fingertip would just reach the button, but then she would have to exert more energy to push it. Her shoulder went into a spasm from the effort, but still she reached. A drop of sweat ran down her forehead, down the side of her face, behind her ear. But still she reached. She must not give up. Her fingertip inched closer. She summoned all the strength of her being and groaned aloud as she touched the button, only to have her hand slide off and drop back to the bed. She dropped her arm in exhaustion. She would try again later.

Main Nursing Station—Wellness Co-op—Computer Terminal

Caregiver No. 42, AKA John Macklin, stood at the main nursing station awaiting his instructions for the day. Apparently the computer had crashed again. The old bat, Betty, who used to run things, had been a real pain, but she sure could make that computer sing. Now Candace, she could get a guy's motor running, but forget it when it came to the computer. Candace shook back her beautiful, thick blonde hair right now and gave him the eye.

"Hi John," she smiled at him.

"Candace, hello, got any orders for me?"

"Oh," she tossed her blonde locks back, "not regarding your patients, but … " She put her hand on her hip and just let him look. He noticed her evenly tanned legs below the hem of her short skirt.

"Really tempting, honestly, I would like to know a bit more, but … " He held his left hand up indicating his wedding band.

"Oh right, you're a newlywed. Hey," she came closer pretending to show him some computer printouts, "that's OK with me. I only need you for, oh, I don't know, say an hour?"

"Yeah, that would be just long enough to get me into major trouble."

"Oh, be that way," she pouted.

He stepped back, face flushed. "Wish they would get this computer going." He glared at Candace. A line formed behind him as the other caregivers arrived for their morning orders, and he had to be careful.

Reinforcements arrived in the form of Garrick Smith and some seedy little guy who Macklin didn't recognize but who turned out to be some computer whiz. It didn't take the two of them long to find the right directions for Gus (the computer's name). The printers began humming, and Candace, her honey blonde hair bouncing, ran from one machine to another collecting the patient files and then delivering them to the appropriate caregiver. Candace paused when she came to Macklin and made eye contact,

"Tempting, but no," he said and grabbed his orders from her. He gave cute Candace one final look. He told himself to forget about any kind of escapade with her as he headed back to his assigned patients. If he hurried, he could do his orders and have time for an extra fifteen at his coffee break. They allowed that now—a little reward for being industrious.

He repressed the nagging thought that rushing the caregivers through their orders was maybe not such a good idea, but what did it really matter? The computer would catch any major snafus. Macklin looked down at his first computer printout:

Andrew, Janis  Rm. 301 Wellness Co-op Baltimore, MD
    Prognosis: Death Certain
    Treatment Level: None Allowed
    Pain Coping Treatment: Meds. Allowed, Code 3
    Date of Discharge: 10/3/2075
    Retirement Home: Valley Home
    Post Death Instructions: Med Tech Center ABS

That last instruction caught John's eye. So Janis had willed her body to the same training school he had attended. John figured her to be one of those intellectual types who still had books (like the ones he saw in some old movie one time). John had worked as a caregiver for ten years—make that ten boring and even tedious years, so he made it a practice to try to guess what his patients had been like when they were young. Old people bored him. He had begun this game when he was reassigned here after having first worked post training in the Pediatric Wellness Center in the former University of Maryland Medical School. What a depressing place. After attempting to improve John's attitude with Z4, the latest mood medicine, the supervisor there had given up and sent him here to work on the hopeless cases. John found this place much easier to cope with and now had his doses considerably lowered. He pushed these "downer" thoughts out of his head like he had been taught by his old supervisor and thought instead of his wife, Gail, and the fun they would have together later after work.

# CHAPTER 2

The house was beautiful in an ancient sort of way. Gail Tilden's observant gray eyes took in the overgrown and untidy yard. She had never lived in a house, only in one of the government provided condos. She followed the brick path up to the front door, tripping at times on the multiple broken bricks. The bushes had grown to eye level height everywhere, and the gnats and bugs to go with so much plant life swarmed around her as she approached the front door. The house itself loomed over her, huge by today's standards, with two windows on the side as well as four in the front. They looked like they actually opened, the old fashioned way. Gail's apartment had just one window as permitted by code, and climate control eliminated the need for it to function like these old things. Gail wondered how the owner of this house had eluded the housing authorities.

Back to her purpose for being here. The structure was certainly large enough and secluded enough for illegal medical activities to be taking place inside. And the law left little room for interpretation. "Medical Care activities may not be carried out anywhere other than in an approved government structure." She took one last look at the punched up file on her laptop computer. She had already studied it in preparation for this inspection, and she had the court permission certificate ready if needed. Inspector Tilden readied herself and rang the doorbell. She couldn't find the intercom outside that most buildings had.

The door opened, and Gail stood face to chest with a man who matched the physical description in her computer file: age 36, brown hair, hazel eyes, oval face, no scars. She stepped back at the suddenness of the door and at his larger than life appearance. His brown hair reminded her of an Italian statue, curly and full. She found the sha-

7

dow of a beard oddly attractive. He just stared back at her, which, of course, made her more uncomfortable.

"Yes?"

"Oh right, yes, I'm Gail Tilden, from the National Medical Review Division of the Government Distribution System."

He looked at her in silence. She smiled uncomfortably. Finally, he said, "You're a government agent?"

"Yes, really, I'm here, um, I'm here because we have had some complaints regarding activities here."

"Really?" His quiet attitude made her nervous.

"Yes, well, I work for them, and I just need to ask you a few questions. If that would be all right with you?"

"I suppose. You want to come in?"

"Um, yes, actually. I have a warrant for that, but, you know, I don't like to bring that up," she said as she followed him in.

They had made it just through the door when he turned abruptly. She almost walked into him. The corner of his mouth twitched slightly. "Of course, you'd rather pretend like you've come for some herbal tea?" She had no response and looked away.

"Whatever. I guess I have to have you in." He stepped aside as he allowed Gail, The Inspector, inside.

Mr. Chambers led her into the living room and the words, old, old money just popped into Gail's head, making her more suspicious than she had heretofore been. One of the characteristics of an illegal caregiver was inherited wealth. She looked around again consciously trying to determine what had made her mind leap to this conclusion. Maybe wallpaper—something she had never seen—made her wonder about him. The old and faded paper as well as the worn fabric on the sofa probably had something to do with her aroused suspicion. There were rugs with old-fashioned floral patterns, and the wood furniture really had a strange effect on her. She had never seen so much wood inside a building before; tables, chairs, a desk in the corner, even what must have been a dining room table—all items whose production was made illegal in 2023 (The Save the Trees Legislation). She noted the empty bookcases. Nobody had those anymore. Mr. Chambers turned and nodded toward a high back, golden damask covered chair. She couldn't resist touching the fabric before sitting down. She hoped Mr. Chambers didn't notice. She resumed her business persona as she sat down. Get a grip, she thought. He smiled at her somewhat condescendingly, Gail wilted again under his stare. Those eyes! They were having an intimidating effect on her, and she could tell he knew it.

"So, what can I do for you?"

Gail took a deep breath, "We received an anonymous tip that someone is giving medical care out of this location, without any government license. My office has sent me to investigate the allegation."

He considered this. "I'd like to see those papers now."

She nodded, and began to reach into her briefcase to retrieve the paper. He quickly put his hand up, grinning, "Stop, I believe you have the proper authority. Just tell me what I need to do."

"Mr. Chambers, I consider this a serious matter." She tried to stay objective, but this man annoyed her.

"I'm sure you do." Silence again. He smiled, "Let's get this over with, so I can go back to work. My accounting work. What makes you and your supervisors think I have done something illegal?" he asked.

"Like I said before, we had a tip. Someone who called saying there was much traffic here. People coming and going at odd hours. Even a few spotted with canes and wheelchairs." Gail paused. She didn't want to press too hard and have the case thrown out because of procedural code violation. "Perhaps if I just ask a few questions, fill out this form for you, and if you don't mind allowing me to look around. Maybe I can clear this up for you, so that you won't be further bothered by us?"

R. Stephen looked at her with squinty, noncommittal eyes. "Good plan."

Gail stood, and so did he. "Ok if I look around now?" He just nodded and shrugged his shoulders. Gail noticed how short she felt next to him. Her five-foot seven self shrunk next to his height of at least six feet. He ran a hand through his tousled brown hair, looked around the room, squared his shoulders and said, "I'll just wait here."

Inspector Gail Tilden opened her car door and heaved her laptop and briefcase onto the seat next to her. After two hours of asking dumb questions that got her nowhere and a lengthy search of R. Stephen Chambers' home, she had found no evidence whatsoever. In fact that was what really bothered her. No thermometer, no painkillers or mood modifiers, nothing in the way of household meds. She had asked many questions about his daily routine and life as an accountant. Now her job would be to check everything out. This was the truly boring part of her job. She knew his irritation with her didn't mean guilt as she knew no one liked having her come in and poke around in their lives and homes. He certainly hadn't been impolite. He hadn't been friendly either—just belittling, as if he knew he could charm her with his looks. Gail decided she would have to go further back in her research of R. Stephen Chambers' genealogy. Most medical offenders had old time physicians in their family history. Gail had already gone back three generations in Mr. Chambers' history and found nothing suspect.

Gail decided to dismiss it all for the moment and picked up her phone to call her husband, John, at the Wellness Center. She needed to hear a welcoming voice and some of that reassurance that John would give.

He answered immediately, "Hi Babe,"

"John. Oh, it's good to hear your voice. How is work? "OK. It's going OK."

"Good, that's good. Mine isn't so great. Not a big deal really and nothing different."

"Your boss on your case again?"

"Actually, no, not this time. Just annoyed with the last client I saw."

"Oh, sorry to hear that."

"They take out their annoyance with the government on me."

"Tell me about it. Totally unfair." John thought of his patients who complained routinely to him.

"Yep. I kept my cool though."

"That's good, Gail. Look I've got to get to my next patient."

"Right. Of course. No time for me."

"Come on, Gail, you know that's not it. Look, when I get home, we'll do something fun tonight, OK?"

She brightened. "Sure, good idea. I'll call Vern and Suzie to see if they can get together."

"Great. I'll cook something up for us. But I gotta go now—you know how they time everything we do including phone calls."

"Right, right. Ok, see you later."

Her car had still not moved. Was she calling the authorities? Was he going to be arrested? Stephen had been watching Gail's car ever since she had finished her so called investigation. Interrogation was more like it. Stephen wondered if he was going to have to go underground like so many others. Apparently, the Underground had a spy in Ms. Gail Tilden's office because two Underground members had arrived with a truck just one hour before the inspector. They had warned him of her arrival and the three of them had loaded all of his medical supplies into the truck. Then they had brought in the computers to help him with his assertion that he worked as an accountant. Where they had come from and where they had gone, Stephen had no idea. They had told him how to behave with the good inspector, and Stephen thought he had done a pretty decent job. There, finally the car moved. Stephen exhaled and sat in one of his grandfather's old maroon leather chairs.

# CHAPTER 3

The muddy water lapped up against the ancient wooden pier that stood overlooking Baltimore's harbor. A school of fish darted near the wall hoping to feed off the algae that had formed on the wet wood. Standing on the pier, Marcie Geck pulled her stained black sweatshirt around her shoulders as the wind came off the water and hit her body. It was a sunny, chilly fall day in Baltimore. People were milling around. Office workers escaped into the sunshine for their lunch hour. Marcie eyed each one looking for her contact. Her hard, mannish face checked each passerby carefully but discreetly. A large denim bag was slung casually over her left shoulder so as not to belie the fact that inside, fifty thousand dollars in large bills were neatly rubber banded together in bundles. With her right hand, she occasionally put her lit cigarette to her lips. The harbor was about the only place left where you could smoke. Marcie, a chameleon, was dressed to deal with the scum she was about to meet. Then, later, when she met her buyers, she would lose the cigarette and dirty jeans for a conservative business suit. Marcie Geck did what she needed to do to survive.

Soon he emerged from the milling nobodies, that slime, Chuck Waller, now with paper sack in one hand and a meatless sandwich in the other. His belly hung way over his belt, white shirt unbuttoned, jacket just barely staying on his shoulders. He sashayed up to her and grinned that Chuck Waller stupid grin.

"Hi ya darlin'. How's it happenin'?"

"It's not. Back off, Chuck and let me breathe. You smell."

Deeply hurt, Chuck took a step back and eyed Marcie up and down. "Say, Geck, the boss says he's got room for you in The Company."

"Just start movin'.'" All this said in low tones so as not to draw attention, the two walked off as if they were old pals.

"Is that the two?" Detective Rufuos King asked as he watched Geck and Waller stroll down the Harborwalk. "Talk about the odd couple." He shook his head and handed the binoculars over to his partner, Sis Leland. She laughed and peered through the lens at the tall slim and chubby squat figures as they walked away.

"Now what?" Officer Leland turned her head and looked at Rufuos. "How much medicine do you suppose is in that paper bag Waller's totin'? You know they're doing a deal."

Rufuos laughed to himself. How did Sis Leland, ex-Roland Park resident, upper cruster, end up on the Baltimore City Police Force? Sis owned those classic good looks that she minimized by keeping her naturally blonde hair extremely short and her perfect figure hidden under her blue police uniform. More important, she was intelligent and, at the same time, deferred to his judgment most of the time. More than he could say of his last partners. Now what to do? During his stint on the Baltimore City Police Force, Rufuos had seen all kind of crime. He had seen heinous violence and its aftermath. The bloodied unrecognizable bodies. The children left miserable and orphaned. The drugs, the gangs, the vandalism and robberies that turned even worse. It was all ugly, and grisly, and through it all, Rufuos tried to remember his own humanity. He tried to remember there was good out there too.

He saw the good in his wife, Stacey, and their three children, in the people he worked with, people like Sis who could be doing some easy desk job rather than risking everything to be on the street. Rufuos was also aware of the amount of white-collar crime out there, even though he had not been involved in the investigations of such crime. Until now. But this wasn't really white-collar crime. He didn't really know how to classify it. Geck and Waller were breaking the law, no question. The money was for illegal drugs, but these drugs were not going to be abused, at least not in the same way that opium and cocaine were. Rufuos knew these drugs were going underground to physicians outside the System. Unlike opium and other derivatives that ruined lives, these drugs were going to do someone some good even though the government said it wasn't allowed. For all he knew, some of his own friends and even relatives may have used the Underground. Heck, if one of his kids was sick and the System cut them off, wouldn't he do something, anything, to find help?

"Let's just follow them, for now. Okay?" Sis who had been quietly watching the twists and turns on Rufuos' craggy, brown face just nodded and the two headed west on Pratt St. on foot at a distance from their suspects.

By the time Marcie and Chuck had made it through the maze of people and stalls in the Pratt Street Pavilion, they had completed their exchange. Marcie walked briskly but not too fast across Pratt Street and north to Charles Street and Mount Vernon Place where the Universal Health Club was located. Marcie Geck walked in the front door and headed directly to the elevator after Melody at the receptionist desk gave a brief nod. As the elevator door closed behind her, Marcie allowed herself to relax just a bit. Chuck Waller wasn't too bad to deal with as brokers go, but you just never knew when government agents might be watching. Actually it was this element of danger that gave Marcie the only real kick she got in life. Marcie had always been rebellious and after leaving the orphan childcare institution where she had been raised and on which she had centered all her hostility, Marcie had transferred all her anger and frustration to the federal government. Others assumed she had a missionary zeal for the sake of those who needed the medicines she carried, but they were mistaken. Marcie Geck drew great satisfaction from the knowledge that she was making her living outside the establishment which had so poorly raised her.

# CHAPTER 4

"Now we knead the dough for a good long while, my doll." Janis, a wide-eyed child of six looked up at her grandmother's capable and substantial arms. She always felt so safe when Yiayia came to visit. And the smells! The house never smelled so good! Always the smell of garlic and olive oil cooking. Baking smells of cinnamon and anisette. After just one day of Yiayia's presence, the wonderful odors permeated the house. Today, they were making bread, Janis' favorite. Yiayia always included her in these activities and gave her important jobs like adding the sugar and eggs or sprinkling the sesame seeds on top when the bread had been braided and was ready to go into the oven. Janis smiled as she thought of the scrumptious taste of the warm finished bread.

Suddenly, an ugly smell intruded the smell of antiseptic, the smell of death. Janis awoke to the reality that this was not the year 2000 but actually 2075. Instead of baking bread in the safety of her grandmother's kitchen, she lay dying a slow death in isolation, trapped in the cruelly titled hospital, The Wellness Co-op in Baltimore, Maryland. No one remotely like her grandmother would be with her as she passed from this life. Disease had transformed her once beautiful body into a shriveled shadow of what it had been. Only a little gray hair left. On good days when Janis could still formulate thoughts, she wondered how she, of all people, had ended up so totally alone. She had never married or had children, but she had always had friends. Unfortunately, her dearest friends had already gone. It was just her and the cat, Apollo. Her neighbor, old Bill Sanderson, had agreed to care for Apollo while she was sick. But she knew and she knew Bill knew (she had seen it in his eyes) that she would not be coming home.

She heard voices outside.

"Hey John, what's happening?" Who was John, Janis wondered as she lay listening.

"Not much. Gotta check on this patient." Janis heard Caregiver No. 42's voice. She hadn't known his name before.

"Man, how long has she been in?" Janis knew her cutoff date was approaching.

"Long time, close to two weeks now."

"Damn! Aren't you sick of her?"

"Hmm. If it isn't her, it'll be someone else. At least I don't have to do much for her. Just get to my break faster."

"How come they're allowing her to be in so long?"

"Dunno. Think she stayed healthy pretty long, so she hadn't used her allotment."

"Isn't she the weird one they've been talking about? You know, the one they call the wizard?"

"Yeah, I've heard the talk. Don't know if it's true. I haven't actually been able to talk with her."

"Don't really matter though, right? She's headed for Death Alley."

Janis froze. Death Alley! She didn't want to go there. She couldn't go there! She'd been there before to visit friends who were dying. She knew they would stop all meds including the pain meds. She already suffered even with the meds they were giving her now. Besides, when she willed her body to science, the government had told her she would never be put in Death Alley. (Well, they called it Pratt Towers.) She listened carefully for John's response.

"You're probably right. She doesn't have any money or connections."

The pain surged again, and Janis could no longer maintain her lucidity. She surrendered herself to just drift and even moan, though no one would hear.

They had put him with patients who couldn't be saved. Old, hopeless, unimportant patients. John knew why. When he had been in pediatrics, he had been well aware that there were cases where hope was dashed because old Gus, the computer, said so and for no other reason than that. A machine! The U.S. Healthcare Distribution System Guidelines did not come right out and say medical care would be cut off, but the government's medical resources could not match the demand for care in the U.S. He remembered Timothy, a seven year old boy who had taken a special liking to him. Timothy's hands had been mangled from birth and could have been corrected with surgery. But a computer decided that no care would be given. A computer! Anger surged in John starting in his gut and moving right up into his throat. John remembered now the day the computer had given him the discharge orders for Timothy. Because Timothy's legs had already been corrected by a very expensive surgery, the allotment for Patient 57yl (Timothy) was already used in its entirety. He would not be entitled to more surgery until he was twelve, unless he was in an accident. John had actually heard rumors of staged accidents, but he knew Timothy's parents would never do something like that. John's head started to hurt. These thoughts only came to him when his blood level of medicine dropped right before his next allowable dose. Take your pill right now, he told himself. His misgiving still sometimes overtook his reason. He knew he had to take his Z4 to keep his job, but he knew it buried him. On the medicine he didn't feel right, he stopped being John and became some other person that his real self kept his eye on, watching but unable to control.

Caregiver No. 42 headed down the third floor with his clipboard filled with his orders for the day. He was feeling better now, since his break, since his pill, oh so much better since his hit. He smiled cynically to himself. Yes, his worries were gone; just run these orders, get your work done, and home you go. He stopped at 301 first.

He would check on the old weirdo, Janis, lying there, practically gone. He went in and took her vitals, thinking all the while about getting home to Gail. He would cook up something for Gail and their friends (well they were really her friends), Vern and Suzie. He frowned down at Janis as she tried to form some word. He pointed to his watch hoping she would understand that her computer orders only allowed him five minutes in her room. His wrist monitor would go off, and he would lose future break time. Her eyes were open now and alert. Pleading eyes, begging him to understand what she was trying to say. He should ignore her, pretend not to notice. He tried hard not to make eye contact.

"Just rest, Janis, don't fight it. Just rest." John said quietly.

"Ra-a-a" Was she calling him Ray? With great effort, Janis pursed her lips together, "Pra-a-a … " It sure sounded like "pray" to John. Startled, John realized her right hand had gripped his shirt as he had leaned over to listen. He gently pried her fingers off his shirt with his right hand and was amazed to discover he was holding her other hand with his left, ever so gently. Was she smiling at him?

Some strange force took control of John now. The patient, Janis, was actually smiling at him. And more miraculously, he smiled back, holding her hand and actually feeling satisfied. No—more than that, something, some emotion that had been alien to him. He had the distinct impression that he felt, well, yes, happy. Not to be confused with high, or mellow or even elated. None of those fit. He was happy being there with some old lady named Janis who he didn't really know. And then the weirdest thing of all happened. Tears were coming down his face. At first, John didn't know what the wet stuff all over his face was. Tears? He tried to remember when he had last cried. He knew it was back at peds (the pediatric duty) when he last had shed tears. He knew this would mean heavier doses of his Z4 if anyone happened in and saw him. He thought bitterly, nothing to worry about. It wasn't like the co-op was crawling with workers. He felt happy and strange and then dangerous. John looked at his wrist monitor. He examined it like it was the first time he was looking at it. It was, after all, only a machine.

Janis felt relief surge through her at the touch of another human being. In another time, she knew she would have been surprised that it was Caregiver No. 42. He always seemed so aloof, so unseeing, but here he was, standing next to her bed, holding her hand, smiling, his brown hair hanging over his gentle eyes. When he had started crying, she had tried to squeeze her hand tighter around his. She summoned all of her strength for this difficult task. Her exhaustion made this almost impossible, but she needed to touch him, so she continued to grasp his hand as her pain worsened from the effort. She felt sorry for John, but she didn't know why. Maybe because he was young. She felt sorry for the new generation. They had only emptiness to look forward to. At least she had had family at one time and some sense of community. She had known the experiences of reading books, and hand writing letters, of sticking your hand into a big bowl of flour and feeling how it defined softness. Kneading dough to make bread and then the glorious smell of the bread as it baked in a conventional oven like the one Yiayia had—the kind they had even before the extinct microwave.

Janis remembered what a difficult child she had been, her mind wandered—all the while she looked into John's eyes. She remembered shaving her head when she was seventeen—all for shock value—she saw that now. She remembered her father's tears over that one. She remembered her shame at hurting him so deeply over such a trivial stunt. Cancer now had taken almost all of her hair. She had no choice about so many things. She thought of her father's tears again as she reached up with her other hand and felt John's moist cheek. She was at her mother's funeral, her own heart broken, in addition she knew, to her dad's. She was twenty years old, a proud willful university student who totally crumpled at the sight of her lifeless mother. She saw that her father had put a gold bracelet on her mother's right wrist. She reached into the casket to turn it so the engraved floral design would show. Her father put his hand on hers as she tended one last time to her mother. In the very same way, John now placed his hand on hers as she unclasped the ridiculous manacle that was used to monitor this person's every move. Janis looked meaningfully at the water cup on her food tray. As if being directed by silent commands, John picked up the cup and removed the plastic lid. He held the cup which was half filled with water where Janis could reach it and watched impassively as she dropped the monitor into the water. Even now she could see the etched words "Property of the U.S. Government" wavy through the water.

Janis looked at the cup sitting triumphantly on the food tray. Her last thoughtful act as a living being. She looked into John's eyes and smiled as comfortingly as possible. She tried to convey to him her last lucid thought "I don't want to live in a world of wrist monitors. I want to die." She closed her eyes and ceased to exist.

# CHAPTER 5

The crisp fall air hit John in the face as he stumbled out of the back exit of the hospital. He looked up at the gray sky. He'd heard it could be blue again only if the government found the money to clean it up. John looked around at all his fellow humans as he headed down Calvert Street. People walked around seemingly content with their lives. But how many of them were? Were any? Just this morning he thought he had a good life. He had been content to do as he was told, to take designated medicines, live in assigned housing, take the job given him, but now he had a very big problem. To someone else it might seem small. Infractions such as destroying government property did result in consequences such as decreased pay and fewer or no promotions, but that was not the worst part. The worst part was losing control over medication if you were on a maintenance program as John was. Yep, ole' Caregiver 42 was headed for the land of the living squash. He wouldn't be dead the way Janis was. He would be a walking, talking, unseeing vegetable. No way around it. He had to escape. He shook with fear as he realized Gail could not be a part of this. Why? Why couldn't he just accept the meds, accept the job? Accept his boring life? John remembered Janis' peaceful face. He wanted that peace now more than anything. His destiny all along had been the Underground. He just hadn't realized it until now.

John headed for the waterfront. He needed to think, to figure out what his next step would be. How had he arrived in this predicament? Running from the U.S. Government, married to an agent in the very department that would be coming after him. John had been at many a cocktail party with his wife and others like her who held underground medical care in great disdain. He had gone along because he really loved Gail, and he thought he could suppress those old altruistic feelings. But, he had failed. He had tried so hard not to care.

"Go along to get along," one of his shrinks had told him. "Pretend."

He followed Light Street down to where the old Harborplace had been. It was now a hangout for the roughest forms of humanity. Instinct told him there had to be a way into the Underground there.

Locker 489-658 at the Universal Health Club was Marcie's home away from home. She punched her code in, the locker door swung open and Marcie pulled out her navy skirt and pumps. In went the jeans and sport shoes. She wanted to look sleek and in control when she met with Matthew Salmund, the president of Universal Health Club. She transferred her stash to a lush leather attaché case and stuffed the denim bag into her locker, then swung the door shut. She headed to the elevator and back down to the lobby where Melody was stationed.

Melody looked up from her magazine, brows raised.

"I'm ready *now*." Marcie said.

"Mr. Salmund will see you shortly," Melody responded glancing knowingly at Marcie's briefcase. Marcie moved to take a seat and then changed direction and strode past Melody still concentrating on her magazine and through the door marked Manager. Melody did nothing.

Matthew Salmund looked up from his paperwork. "Ah, Marcie. In a hurry, are you?"

"I don't have a honey outside my door to help me, Salmund."

Salmund just smiled. "And where would Melody go if she didn't work here?"

"Right you are—helping society."

"Absolutely." Salmund stood up slowly and peeked over his desk at the briefcase Marcie had put on the floor beside her.

"I think you will be pleased with what I have procured for you this time," Marcie said. She reached for her briefcase and placed it on Salmund's shiny steel desk. She sat down opposite him as he began to take inventory of the briefcase contents.

Matthew Salmund wrote nothing down. He only silently read each label on the vials and committed to his memory a list of the merchandise. Satisfied, he reached for his own briefcase next to him on the floor, placed it on his desk and carefully placed each bottle in it.

Tall, very fit, Salmund wore clothes of the finest quality, and his meticulous behavior extended to his surroundings as well as the people who worked for him. Marcie had nothing but contempt for the man. She eschewed the phoniness of dress and surroundings. But she knew how to play his game and, therefore, stood before him trading cold, unemotional glances with him. She had dressed in her most conservative business suit, her straight, light brown hair combed back in a simple, neat style thus separating herself as much as possible from that slime, Waller.

"I am pleased. This is very good work. You have done a fine job as usual, Marcie. Your work does not go unnoticed." Salmund smoothed his graying hair with one hand, though it was perfectly in place, and looked directly at Marcie, "I have something else I would like you to do."

Marcie began to protest that there would be no more supplies coming for at least a week, but Salmund calmly signaled with his hand for her to stop.

"I have a somewhat different type of errand for you. A different type of procurement, if you will."

Marcie simply waited. His patronizing manner had always annoyed her.

"I don't know if I can help or not," she said irritably. "I have already been in here longer than appropriate. I don't believe anyone followed me, but I always like to be cautious."

"Quite right. I will come right to the point." Salmund sat down and leaned back in his luxurious, upholstered chair. (The only one of its type Marcie had ever seen. Where did he get this stuff?) "I am going to give you two addresses. I want you to visit the first using your car and collect a man named R. Stephen Chambers. He will be expecting you. You need only tell him your first name. Take him to the second address. Again, you will be expected. And, that's it. Simple. No Waller or any of his type to deal with. I will pay you an extravagant amount of money. Naturally, this is confidential. You will tell no one. You will write nothing down."

"I take it what you're having me do is illegal?"

"Why should that bother you? It never has before."

"I don't go in for helping criminals," Marcie said, her hostility showing, angry at the thought of doing Salmund's dirty work.

"He is no criminal," Salmund continued forcefully. "This isn't the Black Market," his voice getting louder. Marcie was surprised; she had never seen Salmund display any emotion, not ever, even when she knew he had to be extremely displeased with a delivery. Reacting to Marcie's expression, Salmund paused and calmly continued, "You will find Mr. Chambers different than anyone you have ever met. You will not find him offensive. Nonetheless, I am prepared to pay you more than your usual fee, in cash, of course. You do not have to speak to this man other than to tell him who you are and why you are there."

Matthew took a minute to write something on a piece of paper. Looking up at Marcie, he turned the paper so she could read it. Then he put it through the shredder he kept conveniently behind his desk.

"Oh, I think I can handle your little assignment," Marcie answered, her usual spark returning. Matthew Salmund's demeanor had thrown her off today. In past meetings, they had never exchanged more than a few words. She had always thought of him only in passing and then, only with pure contempt.

"You understand. I care about this."

"I get it. I get it. You will get your money's worth."

"Just get him there. Safely. Discreetly." In a rare move, Salmund walked around his desk to stand too close to Marcie. "I can't emphasize how much this matters to me."

"Really? Interesting. I didn't think it mattered to you how you made your money." As if breaking away from a trance, she shook her head and reached for her briefcase. "Whatever. I'll take care of it. No problem." She offered her hand, and he shook it.

Marcie nodded and left quickly. Melody smirked at her as she left. Once out on the street, Marcie wondered aloud, "What are you getting me into, Salmund?" Jumping into the unknown did not appeal to Marcie, but she had to admit, Salmund had never cheated her out of a single dime. And that alone sure was unusual.

The cold damp wind blew in from the harbor tearing at Sis Leland's perfectly chiseled face as she bought two hot dogs, a large cup of fries and two large coffees, one black for herself and one loaded with cream and sugar for her partner. Laden with lunch, Sis headed back to the car where Rufuos waited with the heater running. As she slid into the front seat the police radio sounded an alert. Rufuos pointed his car in the direction of the Universal Health Club where he and Sis planned to do some questioning after lunch.

"All officers in the vicinity of Pratt St and the harbor, be advised, a low level caregiver has escaped and is demanacled. Thirty-five year old white male, brown hair, brown eyes, 5'11", 170 lbs. Please detain. Caregiver is unarmed. Name, John Macklin."

Instinctively, both officers immediately scanned the area looking for anyone well dressed and clean.

"He's going to stand out down here!" Rufuos said laughing. "We'll let someone else look for him. Let's keep to our original plan." Steering the car expertly with one hand, he was halfway through his hot dog and hitting the fries hard. Sis smiled and then suddenly turned serious as he pulled up to the club.

"There she is!" Marcie Geck looked directly at Rufuos as she stepped off the curb to cross the street. "She changed her clothes, I almost didn't recognize her."

Rufuos returned the passive stare and spoke quietly, "I don't know that I would have known her."

"She sure cleaned up to look a whole lot different than when she went in," Sis said thoughtfully. "Should we follow her or go inside?"

Rufuos groaned. Either way it was going to be a waste of time. He hated this detail. He wanted to go after the real bad guys not political miscreants. Yeah, Waller was slime, and Salmund was slick, and Marcie—well probably everything she did was illegal. He just didn't get that bad feeling about any of them that he needed in order to be motivated on the street.

Noticing her partner's hesitation, Sis decided to make the decision, "Let's follow her. We already questioned the other two and got nowhere. She knows we're following her, but I'd still like to see where she hangs out. And … maybe she'll make a slip?"

"No, she won't," Rufe answered, "but we'll go after her anyway. I think she is up to something." He wiped the leftover grease off his fingers onto one of the napkins Sis had brought and pulled out into traffic. Making a left U-turn, he positioned himself so that he could pick up after Marcie as she came out of the garage.

Suddenly, he jumped as someone tapped his car window. It was Marcie Geck, her face close to the glass. He lowered his window and she backed off just a bit.

"Just thought you'd like to know, I'm not using my car this time. Think I'll head for the subway." She glanced at Sis and headed across the street and down the stairs to the labyrinth below. Rufuos and Sis looked at each other and jumped out of the car to follow on foot.

# CHAPTER 6

John gazed into the muddy, sewage filled water of the Baltimore Harbor. He saw a stranger in his reflection. Someone with no place in the world, no special talents and certainly no special or handsome features. John Macklin faced this truth and thought of how many others were like him, with no defining characteristics. He felt pain and anguish. I know, I know, I'm not supposed to think about it, he thought. Life seemed to be all about repressing feelings. He looked around the dingy, smelly downtown shopping area, once a showplace. Only the most forsaken came. They all looked the same to him, these homeless creatures. They all looked passive and empty, but John knew that could not be true. Each one had to have a story filled with highs and lows, bitterness and grief. Why had he always felt different even while trying to fit in? Pretender. That's who he was, but no more. His rash action had probably already produced a chain of events that would be difficult to stop even if he wanted to. He couldn't apologize for what he did. He had hated his job since forever. He was sorry for what this would do to Gail, his wife. Had he pretended with her also? Could a person who acted his way through life be able to know what his own true feelings were? He searched through his list of emotions the way he had been taught in therapy: fear, anger, joy, happiness, sadness. He searched, but found, to his surprise, he could locate no real sentiments of any kind. Intellectually, he knew that should scare him, but it didn't. If he could just sleep for a while. Sleep and join this group of vagrants wandering and not thinking. The sunlight, warm on his face, invited him. The park bench seductively beckoned. He fell into a sun induced sleep, unaware of the police car passing by.

R. Stephen Chambers dozed on his grandfather's old stuffed couch until the harsh ringing of his phone disturbed him.

"Gather your things, personal such as wallet with ID, and a few changes of clothes. Leave everything else. A car will be there in an hour. We are sending someone named Marcie." The voice was clear and an unknown one to him. He had followed directions to the letter. He stood, checking the window, watching for his ride into the unknown. Stephen knew he'd been lucky so far. Lucky to be able to practice medicine the old way, the way of his parents. He knew he had been alone, but, always being so engrossed in his work, he hadn't missed others. His patients had been his social life, his family, his reason for living. He was worried about them. Who would take care of them if he left? They relied on him for all sorts of advice. He tried not to feel guilty for getting caught. Probably his name just came up randomly on Ms. Gail Tilden's computer. He couldn't even feel anger toward her. She looked as if she knew nothing of the real world. Just did her job and went home. Like a robot. No feelings. That's how he viewed most people out in the world. The person at the grocery store, the repair person, his neighbors—all in a stupor. They couldn't think for themselves. They didn't know what that meant. It was foreign to them. We have elected officials for that. The appropriate government agency would take care of that. We do what people like Gail tell us to do.

There it was, a tan, late model, electric car like the one his neighbors had. A tall, slim woman emerged from the car, dressed in a suit with a no nonsense look about her as she purposefully walked to the door. He opened it immediately and looked at her expectantly.

"I'm Marcie," she said simply. She looked meaningfully at his suitcase, and he responded by grabbing it and a backpack. She said nothing. He followed her to the car. After tossing his stuff into the backseat, he climbed into the front and had barely closed the door when she pulled away, the engine sputtering just a bit. Stephen latched his seatbelt and grabbed hold of the inside handle on the door.

"Should I be scared?" he asked. "The way you're driving, either I should be afraid of the government, or I should be afraid for my life."

Marcie looked at him, "I'm a survivor. I hope you are too, because I don't like being involved with anyone who isn't. I'm not beautiful. I'm not smart the way you must be. I'm just good at taking care of myself. It's what I do. I've been hired to take care of you for a while. Don't be a martyr. Don't be difficult when I tell you to do something. You OK with this?"

He nodded.

"I hope you mean that for real, because as soon as I drove into your neighborhood, I knew this was big. Who are you anyway?"

Stephen looked at Marcie. He'd surmised in the few minutes they had been together that she was self-contained and tough. She had sharp features, a pointed nose, a somewhat pointy chin, silky honey brown hair sensibly cut. Her eyes were light brown and alert though small and set a little too close together. Smiling was probably something she didn't do. But who did anymore? He couldn't remember his father or mother smiling much. Being their only child, he was very close to them. They never sent him to be with the other children at daycare. And when he went to school, they picked him up afterwards even when they still had more patients to see. No, they didn't smile, but they did seem at peace. Looking back on it now, were they? Or did they keep their feelings hidden from him. They weren't cynical. Marcie, and Ms. Tilden, they were most likely both very cynical, the way most people were these days. So who am I, he asked himself. He looked at Marcie.

"Well, don't you know?" she asked him impatiently. "I'm sticking my neck out for a nobody? I don't think so. You're someone."

He sighed and looked at her with surrender on his face. "My parents were Ann Ratin and Zachary Stade." He watched her mouth form an "O" in recognition. She took her eyes off the road to look at him, checking for any sign of deceit. He just gazed back at her with his sad eyes. The eyes of a son who had suffered.

"The two doctors who were killed in the demonstrations of 2049?"

He looked away out the window, "I was ten years old, I've been living alone since my grandfather died last year. My mother's stepfather actually. I took his name, Chambers, legally. That's what my mother wanted. She knew she and Dad were targets. My grandfather raised me, taught me the important part of medical knowledge. I went to State Medical School, of course. But he taught me what was important to know, not the "System Way" they teach in school. We worked together. We've been running a clinic for those who have been told they were entitled to no more healthcare. We didn't want people resorting to the Black Market for their medical care. He died. I continued. It's all I have. We worked quietly, we thought. Somehow my name was picked up, hopefully, only by chance. I'm under investigation. That's why the Underground became involved. I've been getting the medicines from them. I think they are afraid I will lead the government to them, now that I am being investigated, so they sent you to hide me, I suppose. I don't know. They were careful on the phone. I'm worried for you. They used your name on the phone."

Marcie smiled secretly to herself. Who even used their real name on the street anymore?

# CHAPTER 7

Built within the last five years, the Harmony Apartments were in keeping with the architectural style that made Gail feel comfortable. The building was one huge round structure with a large enclosed atrium in the center. Tenants could pay a monthly fee for the use of a small five by five-foot piece of planting square within the atrium area. It meant getting your hands dirty—planting shrubs or flowers was just not something Gail could imagine herself doing. She didn't think John would be interested either. But they both liked their apartment. It had been fun having it decorated. They had chosen greens and browns for the walls and furniture. It was not huge, just a living area, food prep area, bedroom and den. As she entered, she looked around for John. It was time he was home. She had decided to have dinner delivered, and she wanted his input, so where was he? Strange, ever since she had known John, he'd been right on time for everything. She usually could predict his movements, but lately he had seemed withdrawn. Perhaps counseling was necessary. Her friends, Gary and Mattie, laughed at them because they had never been to counseling. Truthfully, Gail thought it odd that John wouldn't go to therapy with her. She knew he'd been treated by therapists in the past. Just about all of her friends had their own therapists. She believed continued marital success depended on therapy.

Her stomach rumbled with hunger. Where was he? She switched on the digital music center on her computer to drown out the quiet. Suddenly, the two tone sound of the phone signaled an incoming call. She flipped her computer switch to receive pictorial monitoring as well as the call. The face of that tech at the Wellness Center, Candace, came on.

"Hi, Ms. Tilden. We're looking for John. He left without turning in his bracelet. Probably just forgot."

"He has a late class, won't be home for another two hours. I'll give him the message." Gail lied. She switched off the phone and sat down to think. "Where have you gone and what kind of trouble are you in?" she whispered to the empty room. "Don't make my father right about you, John." Her parents had warned her not to marry John. He comes from a tech background, she remembered her father saying. He had researched John's computer history and discovered that John had the weakness known as Increased Irrational Sentimentality Syndrome. Gail had overlooked that. John was good looking enough and fun to be with. What more could she ask for? She decided to put it all out of her mind. She moved over to her desk and pulled out her file on Chambers. What a weirdo! Her father ought to be glad she didn't marry someone like that! She smiled to herself at the thought.

John awoke with a start. He sat up and massaged his left shoulder which had stiffened as he lay on the park bench just steps away from the chilly harbor waters. Where could he go besides the Underground? If he could spare the embarrassment to Gail, he would. Did he want to die? It would be an easy task. Sneaking back into the hospital would be a cinch. He could change the stock files on the medicines. He could increase his own meds without consulting his therapist. He could sleep forever.

"So, why don't you?" he said aloud as he leaned over the edge of the harbor and saw his reflection in the polluted waters. "Why not?" He asked himself. He reached into his pocket and pulled out his identifier bracelet. He ran his fingers over the etched word, "Property." He squeezed the bracelet hard in anger hurting the palm of his hand and then released it into the black liquid of the Baltimore harbor below.

A surge of joy energized him! He knew why he couldn't end his life. He finally, for once, felt too good to even contemplate suicide. How bizarre. He felt good! How long had it been? He tried to remember a time when he felt the emotion called joy. He closed his eyes and let the tape in his mind of his life run fast through his brain. He could not find a joyous picture. He smiled when his parents praised him as a youngster. He smiled when he graduated. He smiled at Gail as they took their wedding vows. He smiled when they rented their first apartment. But now he looked in the water and laughed out loud. Staring back at him was a person, someone he had never seen before, someone he thought he could like. He stood up, looked around and headed for the subway.

The smell assaulted his senses as John descended into the dungeon (as the subway was called). He had to get out of Baltimore, and he knew inland was better than toward the coast. Too many patrols there. He struggled to ignore the stench and brushed past the beggars who approached him as he entered the loading stage. West was the answer. He shuffled off into a dark corner to wait for his train.

Stephen was feeling edgy. Could he trust Marcie? Here he was in her rusty excuse for a car traveling west and then northwest, as well as he could tell, with someone he didn't know. They had stopped alongside the highway. Well, what used to be a highway. Now the road was merely a cleared area wide enough for two lanes. The surface was more gravel than pavement after so many years of neglect. Who bothered to come to outcountry anymore?

He watched Marcie. Intent on studying her map, her brow creased in concentration, she was trying to find something or somewhere. She had refused to fill him in on their destination. He figured neither one of them had ever been this far into outcountry. He looked around and saw mostly barren ground covered with dust. An occasional, abandoned house, rickety with age, teetered in the wind. One good shove would topple any of the buildings still left standing.

"How long are we going to keep wandering around out here in the middle of nowhere? How long are you going to keep secret what is happening here? I should never have gotten into this car with you," Stephen said irritably. He was tired and scared of the future. He missed his daily routine, his lab, his patients. But most of all he missed being in charge; here he had no sense of control. He had put his faith in a total stranger.

"Look, I'm all you've got right now," Marcie replied calmly.

"You need me, so just be quiet and let me concentrate. Frankly, I'm wondering what you got me into." Instinct told her she should just dump him here and leave, but she knew she had to follow through, or Salmund wouldn't throw any more work her way. She didn't like admitting it, but she needed Salmund to survive. Jobs that he gave her were saving her from life in the subway. There was no place for Marcie in this world except the place she made for herself.

Chambers looked at her disgustedly and decided to get out and walk around for a while. He headed across the street to an abandoned gas station kicking bits of debris such as cans and papers as he went. He looked around. The area would be quite beautiful if it were not for the degenerating structures that were everywhere. Old buildings, like this gas station, with their ugly signs were decaying into piles of rubble. He sat down on a rickety old bench and soon began to doze. The warm sun lulled him into a relaxed sleep. He could hear a voice calling to him. He started forward as he awoke. Marcie called to him. She ran toward him pointing back down the road in the direction from which they had just come. He took a look in the direction she indicated. A man in dirty bedraggled whites came toward them. He waved his hands in the air and shouted something that became "Wait!" as he drew closer.

Marcie looked at Chambers, "Well, what should we do? We could make it to the car and leave. He would never be able to catch up."

Chambers looked directly into her eyes and said, "Should we be afraid of him? I mean, look at him. He's dirty, his clothes are a mess. He's stumbling along. How can he hurt us?"

"Maybe he's a government agent, disguised. He could be," she replied.

"Maybe you are a government agent."

"Oh please. No way would I be out here with you in that hunk of metal I'm driving."

"Right. I guess we all have our secrets."

"Hey, are you going to whine all day or what? I can see the guy's eyes already."

Sure enough, Chambers could make out his face. "I don't think he's the government. He doesn't even have a car. He looks desperate and even confused. Kind of pathetic really. He may really need help."

"Hmmm. He looks like trouble to me." She walked over to her car, reached into the glovebox and withdrew a pistol which she held in her hand, arm hanging down at her side. After a quick glance at a stricken Chambers, she turned to face the stranger.

Chambers backed away in fear, "A gun! You have a gun?!"

"Yeah, Mr. Doctor. I've got a gun. So what? You think anyone is going to know it out here? Anyone is going to care? And what if he has a gun?" She nodded in the direction of the oncoming stranger. Worried about what she might do, Chambers stepped in front of Marcie and confronted the disheveled man as he approached.

"What are you doing out here?" Chambers said.

The man, obviously tired, gave him an appraising stare, then did the same with Marcie as she moved from behind Chambers, eyes settling last on her gun. He stumbled back when he saw it, right up against Marcie's car. Visibly shaken, he pleaded, "I just need a ride to the next town. My car broke down a ways back."

"When? When did it break down, what time?" Marcie asked suspiciously.

"I don't know," he said as he slid along Marcie's dirty car away from where Chambers and Marcie stood. "Who are you people?" the man demanded. He took a deep breath and blurted out, "Are you with the government?"

Marcie glanced over at Chambers and looking back at the man said, "No, are you?"

"Not hardly," came the reply.

"How can we believe you?" Marcie persisted.

The man said nothing, just kept staring at her. Then he said, "How can we believe each other?"

"Do you know the Underground password?" Chambers said with a take-charge attitude.

Eyeing Chambers thoughtfully, Marcie looked at the strange man and said the password opener. Surprisingly, he gave the proper response. How had he gotten it, and who was he really? Still a bit doubtful, Marcie said, "We'll give you a lift. Where are you going?"

"I don't know."

"Oh, great," Marcie groaned and gave Chambers an accusing eye. "Well, do you know your name?" she asked.

"John Macklin"

"OK. John, this is Stephen and I'm Marcie. That's all you need to know. Is there really a car? Should we go back to get your gear?"

John crumbled under her stare, and then decided not to lie, "No. No car. No gear."

Marcie smiled to herself. Right, an innocent guy. "Are you on drugs?"

"Hah!" John blurted out. A wave of nausea overcame him. "Actually, I am in withdrawal."

"Oh great. Last thing we need is a drug addict."

"No! No!! My drugs were legal." John could see she didn't believe him.

"Right, sure."

"No really, legal. In fact I was *required* to take them. See that's why I'm in trouble! You know, I'm not on the ... " He turned and ran to the other side of the care and heaved.

"Here, let me take a look at him," Chambers said. After checking John's pupils, he said, "Has all the signs of it."

"Ha! You see?!" John doubled over again as another wave of nausea hit. He laughed and choked and finally fell into a heap on the ground.

"Oh, this is just great! Now what do we do?" Marcie turned away in disgust.

Chambers peeked over the car at John now lying on the ground. "I think he's harmless. He certainly can't hurt us in the condition he is in."

"I refuse to touch him. You want to bring him, you get him up and into the backseat."

"So, something you can't deal with." Chambers smirked and turned to help John. "Come on then." Chambers said gently to John.

"See, he's nice," John said as Chambers dragged him past Marcie. John crawled into the cramped backseat and tried to relax. The rolling in his stomach had settled at least for the time being. How long had he been on drugs? Years. His body sure knew it. At least he was safe for the moment. The other two got into the car.

Marcie took one last look at her map, folded it, and said, "I've got it, I think." She looked down the road and glanced briefly at Chambers next to her and then Macklin in the backseat. "I think I know where we're headed now. I just don't know what kind of building we're looking for. But I'm sure we'll find it. Then you will be safe at least." Stephen nodded noncommittally. Marcie turned around and looked at John who cowered in the backseat, "I don't know about you."

John tried to disappear. Who was this woman? Well, he had no choice. He could not keep going as he had been. Marcie started up the engine, pulled onto the "road" and continued to head north. Soon they were out of Maryland and into Pennsylvania. John tentatively laid his head back against the dirty, scratchy seat and tried to rest. With his eyes open, of course.

# CHAPTER 8

Dr. Marilyn Shakira took a look outside. Usually her work kept her too busy to even think about what happened outside, but today was different. The excitement had spread through the hospital. A new doctor would arrive soon. Someone who had been making it in the city. Marilyn had so many questions for him, both medical and social. What was happening in the real world? In outcountry, little news filtered in. They knew only what came through on television and computer. Since the media only spread propaganda, people like Shakira had to depend on personal accounts that came from arriving patients. Most of the time, she was happy to be here away from it all, doing what she had always wanted to do.

The commune sustained itself for the most part. The major exception was the medical supplies. All brought in by some elaborate system. She knew it involved theft from the city health suppliers, but she had to believe this was the only way true medical knowledge could survive. Underground organizations historically always had to break some rules. The current Underground health system broke all government rules for healthcare delivery. But they existed to fill a need. Most of the personnel here were like herself. They had started working for the federal and state medical programs, but when the government squashed competent healthcare delivery, many caregivers, after becoming discouraged, found themselves one way or another in a place like this, called a commune to all outward eyes, a farm, but in reality an Underground hospital and clinic. They all had friends or colleagues who had been imprisoned or killed in various purges in the name of the U.S. Healthcare Distribution System Act of 2045. Their connection with each other was the computer, networked only with other Underground hospitals and clinics, but always susceptible to outside intervention. Still, they couldn't keep up with all the new diseases and treatments out there. Occasionally a hacker would get into the federal computers and access new information. It was helpful, she had to admit, to see what the government doctors were doing. This new doctor arriving today could give then some new insights. She had heard he'd operated an underground medical practice of his own for a long time.

An abrupt shift in the appearance of the road occurred as Rufuos and Sis's police cruiser reached the Baltimore Metro limits. The road was not only overgrown but it was rife with potholes. After they hit one of the worst yet, Sis looked over at Rufuos behind the wheel and said, "Pull over for a minute." Rufuos pulled carefully over into the overgrown brush that was covering what was once the shoulder of the road.

"Is this really worth it? I mean we're not going to be heroes over this. Marcie can keep us running after her forever. We're going to have to stop sometime. Is it going to come down to who runs out of gas first?"

"Yeah, and pretty soon we'll be out of our area of jurisdiction. She is headed for outcountry. There's nothing out there. Look, we already chased her all through the dungeon, only reason we found her was luck once we came topside, but she can lose us. She may even head back to the city. She'll have to come back eventually. She's a city girl. Someone will pick her up. Besides we don't even know who that is with her. He doesn't look like a bad guy though. What do you think?"

"I think I'm tired and hungry—add disgusted to that. I need to go to another city where stupid stuff like this doesn't happen."

"NSP—No such place," they both said together and laughed.

"Let's see if I can get turned around without hitting a pothole, and let's give Salmund a visit. I'm just aggravated enough to bother him a bit," Rufuos checked his rearview mirror before making the turn.

"Okay by me, anything but this boredom. I'm going crazy here," his exasperated partner replied.

Because of the life that was chosen for him by his parents, Chambers had been taught early to trust no outsider. Realizing that their son had no siblings, his parents worked hard to instill a sense of independence (not a popular concept at the time) in him as a youngster. His parents prized self-reliance above other virtues. Now, stuffed into a car with two people he didn't really trust in an unknown environment, Chambers began to question whether he should have left the city. Marcie appeared to be a courier. Beyond that he knew nothing about her, but had spent the first hours with her trying to guess what she was all about. The backseat passenger seemed a more human person though he also had revealed nothing of his life. Was he safe out here in the middle of nowhere with two strangers? Marcie had mentioned survival. He figured desire was the first attribute needed in a survivor and he certainly had that characteristic. She said she did too, but he suspected they were very different in their reasoning. He tried to remain calm, but he couldn't help shifting in his seat restlessly.

"What's the trouble?" Marcie asked as she observed him move around in the passenger seat. Over and over again for the last hour. "Don't worry, I'm not going to let anything happen to you or our new friend in the backseat," she said with a glance in the rearview mirror. John was sitting upright with a timid look on his face. "What's your story?" she said to John's reflection in the mirror. "How did you end up out here, and where are you going?"

Chambers turned in his seat and stared at him. He wanted answers also. After all, the guy hadn't said two words since he had gotten into the car. He sat, shriveled into the tiny backseat. The fellow inspired sympathy at least from Chambers. Geck didn't look like she had a sympathetic nerve in her body.

Chambers took another look back at John and then turned to speak to Marcie, "What are you going to do with him?"

"I don't know. You have suggestions?"

"We could take him with us. He might be useful." Turning back to John, "What do you do?" John looked at him thoughtfully, then opened his jacket so the label imprinted on his shirt, "Caregiver No. 42" was visible. Chambers stared at the blue letters, then slowly shifted his gaze to John's face. John looked apologetic. Chambers turned around, and just stared ahead.

"What? What is it?" Marcie asked sensing big trouble. "What does he do?"

Chambers looked her way, "He's a caregiver with the System." He looked into her eyes with intensity and meaning. "A Government

Healthcare System Tech. That's what he is." Marcie brought the car to a careening halt. Both she and Chambers turned to look at John who fidgeted and avoided eye contact.

"Hey!" Marcie used her harshest tone. "What are you up to?"

"Up to?" Now John looked up pleading. "Wait a minute. You are afraid of me? Me? That's a total laugh. I'm nothing. Nothing to anybody. I have nothing. And hey," a defiant tone entered his shaking voice, "what's wrong with being a caregiver? You don't like us? Why?"

"If you can't answer that on your own, I guess we're safe." Marcie made her decision about this guy. He looked harmless. He acted lost. And he might be worth something. "All right guy, John, whoever you are. You've got to come clean with us or we're leaving you right here. And I don't know when the next car will ever come by. We haven't seen one for the last fifty miles, so tell us everything. We need to know all."

As John's eyes rested their gaze on his left wrist, so did the eyes of Chambers and Geck.

"I took it off."

"What? Took what off?"

"My wrist locator. I took it off. I ran away. I couldn't do it anymore. I couldn't do it. Couldn't watch 'em die. All day long. Dying people. No help. No care." He spoke rapidly now. "Medicines cut off. Couldn't do it." John dropped his face into his hands and sobbed quietly.

"What a coincidence, another healthcare professional. This is just great. Salmund, this is all your fault."

"Who is Salmund?" Chambers asked.

Marcie shook her head disgustedly. "Nobody you need to know. He's just the guy that got me into this mess. And now look," she took a breath. "I'm stuck with you, and I'm stuck with him." She turned her whole body now, got up on her knees, still in the driver's seat and stared at John. John's hands shook, and he shrugged. What a scary woman. "You have nothing to say for yourself, right? No idea about anything." Marcie sighed and turned back, sitting in her seat once again. Marcie looked at Chambers. "What do you think? Is he honest?"

Chambers nodded. "Don't know about the honesty part, but I don't think he will hurt us. Bring him with us."

Oh, this was just great, John thought. I'm with two people who don't seem to like each other very much. They certainly don't like me. And what about me? I'm just headed for another disaster.

While they bickered between themselves, John took the opportunity to carefully turn and look back down the road he had just walked. His tension eased a bit when he realized no one was coming. He dropped back into the fetal position that gave his stomach some relief. With any luck, the motion of the car would put him to sleep. Out of habit, he reached into his pocket looking for his pill container. He brought it up to his face. Empty. Right. Sleep. The only hope for him right now.

# CHAPTER 9

Reverend McClaren stepped back from the pulpit of St. Luke's Lutheran Church. He looked at his liver spotted hands now sprinkled with white paint. The paint on the pulpit would be dry by Sunday for sure. Being a pragmatist, Reverend McClaren saw nothing wrong or even demeaning about opening a can of paint and sprucing the place up a bit. His church had many financial needs; one needed to prioritize. It seemed silly to pay someone to do something he could do with his own two hands. People gave what they could, and he certainly had a congregation he was proud of. Of course only his lay leaders knew about the "healing connection" mentioned in the church budget. The rest thought it referred to the special healing service he himself led each Wednesday evening. He wished he could tell them all, but perhaps this was the Lord's way of teaching him humility. Pride was always difficult for McClaren to overcome or overrule. Still, he knew what he did was important and the work that God wanted him to do.

His church linked sick people with the help they needed. One more step for the government to have to make to find the medical Underground. McClaren believed in the purpose of this church as a cover to protect the hospital it housed in addition to the sanctuary. No one (on the wrong side) had ever made the connection. McClaren carefully wiped his hands on his rag dipped in turpentine and rubbed the paint off of his hands. He didn't think his guests would mind his dress. Denim overalls were pretty much what everyone wore in outcountry. He decided to go get some of Marilyn's lemonade and sit on the porch of the parish house to wait.

Once comfortably seated, McClaren's head, covered with thick wavy white hair, fell forward as the morning's physical activity caught up with him. The forward motion of his head causing him to awaken. As he squinted against the sun, he spotted movement on the horizon.

Across the barren field he spied a gray small car kicking up dust as it traveled nearer. He quickly got up, ran over to the church entrance and hollered "Someone's coming! Don't know for sure who yet … " He took a few steps forward again trying to make out how many were in the car. Marilyn soon joined him and they both struggled to see if the expected guests were indeed in the car.

"I think I can see three. There were only supposed to be two," Marilyn knit her brow as she became worried. "What do you think?"

"Well, my Marilyn, we play it cool, as they used to say. We use the old married story 'til we're sure." He looked at her affectionately. "Why don't you make an honest man out of me and marry me? Then I wouldn't be forced into lying. You know I am a man of the cloth."

Marilyn put her arm around McClaren and smiled contentedly. "You're too good for me," she replied.

"Aw c'mon, I could bring you around!"

"Shh! Hush up now. Here they come. There *are* three. We'd better be very careful."


Marcie did a double take when she saw the church. "That's not supposed to be there. There's supposed to be a factory according to the map Matthew gave me."

"Look! We're tired and apparently lost. Let's talk to those people and see if they can help us." Chambers said.

Marcie steered the car up to the front of the church, put the car in park, and turned to her two passengers. "Stay put," she said with a quick glare at John. John felt himself melt under her gaze. What had he gotten himself into? He could be home right now with Gail having … having what? One of those same vegetarian meals that she insisted they order, and then maybe if he was really lucky, she might deign to have her version of sex with him during which she constantly gave him orders. Then sleep and back to the "factory," which is how he had come to think of the Wellness Center. This woman, Marcie, definitely made him nervous. But the other guy seemed OK. At least they had one thing in common, their disdain for The U.S. Government Healthcare Distribution System.

"Don't worry. Don't worry. Trust me, trust me, I'm not going anywhere and I won't say anything."

Marcie took in everything about him, and he instinctively knew it. He couldn't hide his insecurity from her like he did with Gail.

She took a quick look at Chambers who simply shrugged and said with a bit of a grin, "I'm yours."

She then gave Macklin a stare and as she opened her door to get out said under her breath, "Trust me, right? Trust? Forget it fella, I don't trust."

Always she had to do everything herself. Marcie slowly got out of the car and walked over to where McClaren and Marilyn stood.

"Howdy stranger," McClaren said. Marilyn just smiled sedately as Marcie looked the two of them over noticing the casual way Marilyn had her arm on McClaren's shoulder.

"I think we're a little lost," Marcie began. "We're looking for a factory. I think it's called High Resolution. They make lenses there. Do you know of it?"

"We thought there was to be two of you." McClaren answered.

"What do you mean?"

"Young lady, you just gave us the sign. I'm very big on signs."

"I don't know what you're talking about. Who are you and who were you expecting?"

"Why you, young lady. We've been expecting you and *one* of those fellas. Not two. That's why we've been a little standoffish. I still think you've got to explain yourself a little." Marilyn nodded in agreement.

Marcie felt confused; she felt distinctly confused—one of the worst possible ways for her to feel. "I don't get you, mister. I don't know you."

"Of course you don't. You're not supposed to. You're supposed to show up with one, not two riders; then we do the rest, you see? You're not supposed to have two people with you. So you've got to do some explaining before we move from this spot."

Marcie looked back at the dusty car and her two worn out fellow travelers. "Actually I don't know how you know it, but I started out with one. The one in the front, the scruffy looking one. He's supposed to be with me. The other one. He's dirty and scruffy. Well, we just don't know what to do with him. We kind of just picked him up from alongside of the road. I guess we thought he had an honest face or that he was kind of helpless." Marcie ended feebly. Damn that Chambers for convincing her to pick up that mess of a man, Macklin. She knew how stupid she sounded.

Marilyn could be silent no longer. "Do you realize what you've done? You've endangered the whole program."

Marcie didn't like her tone. "How do you two know anything about the program? I just wanted to ask for some directions. Who are you?"

"Oh, no lady, that ain't the way it works. You tell first. Who sent you?" Marilyn folded her arms and waited.

Back at the car, Macklin grew more nervous by the moment.

"What do you think is going on? And where are we headed anyway?" Macklin asked as he watched Marcie shift her weight from one foot to the other.

"I don't know," Chambers said slowly, "I just don't know." He glanced back at the hitchhiker. "Just keep still and be glad we gave you a lift. I have a feeling you're turning out to be trouble for us."

"Here she comes!" Macklin said excitedly, happy to turn Chambers' attention away from himself.

Marcie had a troubled look on her face as she returned to the car. She opened the door and sat down and said nothing.

"Well, what's the problem?" Chambers asked.

Marcie turned and looked pointedly at Macklin who looked away. Then she turned to Chambers and said, "I never should have listened to you. I don't know why I did. I know better than to rely on anyone else." She breathed heavily and looked straight ahead. "They're calling my supervisor to check me out. They are concerned about our additional guest."

Time passed. Marcie and Chambers dosed in the front seat, but John couldn't relax. He wished he had had the sense to bring some medicine with him. He was finally able to sit up.

"Look!" Macklin yelled jarring the two awake. He leaned forward excitedly and pointed to the Reverend and Marilyn. "They're coming over!"

Marcie followed his glance and lowered her window as the two came over to talk.

"We've decided to keep you," The minister said.

"What about him?" Marcie indicated John with a nod to the backseat.

"We're keeping him, too. He apparently needs us even though he may not know it." All eyes turned to Macklin who indicated his innocence with a shrug of the shoulders.

"Macklin, out of the car. Don't talk."

"I'll keep an eye on him," Chambers had already gotten out of the car and came around to Macklin's side. He felt sorry for the guy.

John's knees barely held him as they walked across the dry dirt to the porch, which led into a church.

# CHAPTER 10

The church had the dusty, dank smell of disuse although the minister insisted they had regular services there. No lights were on; the only source of light was through the windows located high on either side of the building. The minister led the way followed by Marcie, Stephen and John. Marilyn brought up the rear, locking the outer doors as they entered the sanctuary. They followed the minister to a door located next to the pulpit. He pulled open the door revealing a circular staircase leading down to what John presumed was a basement. John stalled. Where were they taking him? Chambers nudged him forward and down. He had no choice but to go along. John reached for the banister, followed closely by Chambers.

First there was light! Blindingly bright! John closed his eyes and then slowly opened to just a squint. Once able to see again, John discovered something very different from a basement. He suddenly found himself in the midst of all sorts of activity. If John didn't know better, he would have thought he was in the middle of the University of Maryland Hospital Center. He looked over at Chambers coming up behind him and noticed his mouth hanging open in awe.

So this was the Underground! He had heard of its existence through his wife's work, of course, but he hadn't really believed it could be this organized. Gail had never talked to him about how Underground healthcare was administered. Of course, she wouldn't have. No one was supposed to know about it. But now. Here it was!! He certainly hadn't expected to find a hospital in the basement of a church.

The large area was divided into a network of halls with many rooms, some connecting. As they walked down the center hall, they looked into the different rooms noticing various types of activities in each one. The minister didn't talk; he just led them on until they finally entered a small office containing only a desk and two chairs. Reverend McClaren indicated they should all enter. Marcie and Chambers sat while Reverend McClaren leaned against the small metal desk. Marilyn pulled the door shut and remained standing next to John.

"Welcome to St. Luke's Hospital, your new workplace, Dr. Chambers and," he turned to John, "yours also. We're happy to have you on board." McClaren formally reached forward and shook Chambers' hand and then John's.

Marcie took a moment to study John Macklin. Ever since they had entered this building, she had noticed a decided change in his demeanor. Suddenly, no more slouching, head high, he seemed interested in everything going on. No longer did she feel he was dependent on her. He seemed right at home. In fact, he asked the first questions.

"How do the rationings work here?"

"Rationing?" Reverend McClaren replied.

"I'm sorry. Am I being too blunt? You look surprised."

Had he offended the minister?

"No, no, not at all. I guess I have to admit I'm a little surprised. You do understand this is an Underground Hospital—not just literally. Rationing? Rationing is a big part of the reason we exist. We want everything to be above board here except, of course, we can't be open with the outside world. You see the difference here is focus. We focus on taking really good care of our patients and holding on to the medical knowledge that took centuries for humans to accumulate."

"For example," McClaren picked up a strange object. "Are you familiar with this?"

John shook his head no.

McClaren turned to Chambers, "Dr. Chambers, do you know what this is?"

Chambers smiled and reached for the long rubber tubing that had a metal disk at one end and made a "Y" at the other, with earpieces on the end.

"My grandfather had one of these, and I have one just like it with my things." He put the earpieces in his own ears, walked over to John, and placed the disk gently under John's shirt and listened. "Hmmm, sounds good. Would you like to listen?"

"Sure, but what is it?"

"This is a stethoscope. For listening to a patient's heart."

Chamber answered. He then put the earpieces on John so he could hear for himself.

McClaren smiled and continued, "A simple invention really, but so useful. Of course back in the late 90's and early part of this century, the feeling in medical training facilities like the one you attended, John, was that technology could do a better job than the doctor using a stethoscope."

"Don't get me wrong. I am not opposed to new knowledge. I just am deeply worried about losing the information we had already." McClaren stopped suddenly, and turned to John.

"So young man, what do you think?"

"Cool, very cool." In fact, John could barely contain himself. But then he remembered. "So how can you afford to take care of all of your patients without any limits?"

"Oh, yes, quite right. Thank you for bringing me back to that. Yes, rationing. We don't do that here. Here Dr. Chambers will be making the decisions. And John, you will contribute to these decisions. You will have time to talk with the patients. You will help Dr. Chambers and Dr. Shakira and our other doctors to evaluate the needs of the patient." He smiled and walked over to John. He tapped him on his head. "We will wake up your brain." He stepped back and studied John for a while.

John felt his face turn red as the attention turned to him. He didn't know what to say.

"You're going to have to choose, you know, young man," the minister said. "It won't be easy. When I called to check you out, our informants told us about the work your wife does. I want you to think about the choice you will need to make."

John took a breath and looked at each one, in turn, in the room. "I'm thinking I already kind of did that."

"Really and how was that?"

"Yeah," Marcie enjoined, "how was that?"

John looked at her finally and then to McClaren, "I've already violated so many laws, I've lost track. I'm not like you people. I've never done anything like this before. I don't even know why I did it or what made me do it. But I'm glad. Ecstatic really that I did it. I just can't handle watching people die who could be saved. Watching people suffer. People can't help it if they are born with lots of health problems." He suddenly remembered, no pills! It had been six whole hours since he had thought about taking a pill. He couldn't remember when that had ever happened. The others were still watching him.

Chambers then said, "Show us some more, Reverend McClaren." Everyone's attention turned from John, and he could breathe again.

"I'll take Dr. Chambers around; I have loads of questions for him," Marilyn said. John watched as Chambers immersed himself in a discussion on patient care and triage techniques with Marilyn.

Marcie and McClaren turned to look at John. Marcie then turned to Reverend McClaren and, indicating John with a nod of her head, said, "Now what do we do with him?" John timidly took the chair Chambers had vacated.

"Believe it or not, John is going to stay with us," McClaren responded.

"Hey, are you talking about permanently?" John asked. "Maybe I should go home? What about my home and all my stuff? And I need to at least talk to Gail."

"Home!" Marcie turned on him and said wickedly, "You don't have a home."

McClaren put his hand lightly on Marcie's arm to silence her. He then turned to John and spoke calmly, yet forcefully, "You go home, and you'll be imprisoned for life, either in a holding facility or a hospital. What difference will it make? Your wife! She's on the other side. You're with us whether you know it or not. There's no going back. You know too much, and you're no longer useful to the System you seem to still have some loyalty to. We know all about you. You don't realize it, but you belong with us. Our people on the outside know what happened to you. They know where your sympathies are. In here, you can be of use. We won't treat you as if you are a robot the way you have been in the past. You will provide real nursing care to our patients."

John could say nothing, stunned into silence. He had never known a minister before, but McClaren's strength still surprised him. And scared him a bit. But he also felt excited, even exhilarated about the idea of really contributing to some of the decisions for the patients. What about Gail? Would she really care that he was gone? They didn't have kids and she could get a quickie divorce. She would probably think that made her cooler. He reached down to his pockets looking for his pills. Then he realized. He could not return for his nighttime dose. He thought about asking for some medicine. Something internal said wait. I can do this. I can make it without the pills.

He felt McClaren's watchful eye on him again, so he decided to risk being without the meds. "Can you show me around?"

"Of course," McClaren answered. "Marcie, why don't you join us? Might do you good to know how the meds and supplies you procure help."

"I guess I don't need to leave just yet." She thought for a minute. "Sure, why not?"

"Let's go then," The three of them walked downstairs to the hospital and strolled slowly down the hall. Patients were on both sides with only curtains dividing them.

"How do you keep up with the Government System's quality of care?" Marcie asked.

The minister looked at her, "You've got to be kidding! The System may have fancier buildings, my dear, but their care is given by techs, you know, like the one you picked up by the side of the road." He smiled gently and apologetically at John. "Here we train doctors and nurses, and they take care of the people. Our problems are shortages of meds and equipment. I know you are a huge help there, Marcie. We actually are getting more doctors than we need for this site. There is talk of developing another location. Need for our services increases when the Government System cuts the choices people have. What can the average person do?" He stopped abruptly and looked intently into Marcie's eyes. "Make no mistake about it. We are not the Black Market. We subsist on private donations only, cash of course. There is no other crime connected to us other than breaking the laws that the System has set up to withhold competent medical care from people. We self-regulate. Our doctors are the best, not only in terms of giving care, but also of teaching others. We have a whole network of physicians who share information. I don't think you've been able to see that. I don't think I'll be compromising our system by telling you that they do it through the newsline. The information is encoded of course. Physicians today have their own binary language, which they use to exchange the most up to date medical techniques. All this and we don't turn anybody away. Except for system investigators of course. So, you see, Marcie, your work enables us to do our work. Oh, there are Marilyn and Dr. Chambers. Let's go watch, shall we?"

Marilyn and Stephen stood on either side of a patient's bed. Marilyn read off the list of symptoms to Stephen and he began his physical examination of the patient.

"You see," Reverend McClaren said to John and Marcie, "the doctors here take the time to question the patients and, through listening to the patient as well as examining the patient, the doctor arrives at the proper diagnosis. Of course, the government has relegated physical diagnosis to machines. Good patient care depends almost entirely on an accurate diagnosis involving not only equipment, but a doctor's judgment based on prior case studies.

Chambers thrived in his element. He had forgotten how isolated practicing medicine away from a hospital was. The prospect of helping the healthcare workers here catch up on the latest medical technology while still using the ancient methods of diagnosis energized him. Marilyn had already introduced him to one of her more complicated patients and he had begun a diagnostic examination while Marilyn watched intently.

# CHAPTER 11

The Star Line had fast become the foremost national news agency. The agency prided itself on being the first to put the latest crisis or news event online. The new software allowed for the fastest verification so that the stories were 65% accurate—the highest rate of any online organization. Reporters vied for the limited jobs available. A stint with Star Line made anything possible for its employees. To be first on the story meant often being able to sell, under the table of course, at least a portion of the information. Paul had risen rapidly to be one of Star Line's top reporters. He had already made two very profitable sales of information (unknown by his superiors, of course). Certainly a man in a hurry, Paul worked hard to present the news.

Paul prided himself on his trim figure—something he worked at regularly, one of the reasons he frequented Matthew's health club. He also took pride in his ability to hide his real motivation from just about everyone.

As he stood outside Matthew Salmund's office after one of his workouts, Paul pondered the world of coincidences. Matthew and he had been in college together. They had never agreed on anything, and yet, here they were on the same side of this health thing. Matthew's point of view was more about people getting the care they needed whereas Paul recognized his own interest as one of constitutional freedom (well, and the money he made providing a circuit for the docs didn't hurt either). Funny. They disagreed about so much. Matthew was actually for socialized quality medicine, and Paul wanted the whole thing broken wide open with total market freedom for the doctors. But on one thing they were clearly together—the current government system did not work. Anyone politically connected could get the most up to date care and medicines – those without such avenues fought over the leftovers—either places like St. Luke's or, far worse, the Black Market.

And of course the other thing connecting them was Christiane. His stomach still turned every time he thought of her. Her skin so fresh, her spirit so full of promise. She was going to be a lawyer. Her hair long and thick tossing on an autumn day. And then. Her end. So lonely, so desperate. Matthew and he finally uniting after being rival suitors. Trying to get her into a wellness center. Being turned down because her case was hopeless. "They wouldn't even try," he thought bitterly as he remembered the various healthcare workers involved in Christiane's case. We didn't even know about the Underground back then. If only she had had a chance. If only they had been connected in some way to the Underground. Of course, they had no money to speak of. They were all students. He and Matthew never talked about Christiane. Ever. But they both knew she was still the motivating force for both of them. Paul tried really hard to forget how she looked that last time. She had cut her hair off in a fit of depression over the pain she was feeling. Her complexion was ratty and colorless. Her body withered to just bones protruding through her now wrinkled skin.

Years later when Matthew had come to him asking for help for the Underground, no one even mentioned Christiane. She was in the room though. Right there looking at them, still tossing her head trying to pretend she felt fine.

Paul said, "Yes, whatever you need." He didn't have to think about it. In fact he found himself constantly searching for ways to channel his guilt. The cloud that hung above him never went away. The guilt over not saving her or at least freeing her from her pain claimed a portion of his brain. He knew Matthew had called him over today because he needed something. But that was all right with Paul. Every activity gave him relief from the desperation he felt. He could never divorce himself totally from the memory of Christiane. He needed a path—a way to get out from under that cloud.

"Welcome, Paul."

"Hey Matthew, how are you?" Paul entered Matthew's office and sat down. Matthew stepped around him to close the door.

Matthew wasted no time with pleasantries, "We're experiencing shortages with our medicines. We need more access to drugs. But also the next step, if the Underground is to continue to keep pace with the outside system, is we need access to the biggest and best medical libraries. Is there a way we can tap into their systems via your circuits? The docs are telling me this is vital to the survival of proper medical techniques." Matthew began pacing around the room and around Paul.

Paul waited until Matthew had made a full circle around the room and back to his desk. Then he said, "I'll see what I can do. I'm going to have to go back in at night and work at the main frame computer." Paul paused and looked straight at Matthew. "I'll take care of it. Tell the docs they'll get their info. With the drugs, I just don't have the know-how. Is there someone else you can call on for help? How about Marcie? She seems resourceful."

"She's out of town right now. I miss her, I can tell you that. She's my most reliable procurer. She knows the dealers, and she gets me whatever I need. I'm going to have to call her back in. She is in out-country making a delivery." Did Paul detect a wistful tone in his friend's voice? It had been a long time since Paul had noticed any softening in Matthew's face.

But all he said was, "I'll see what I can do about getting into the medical library mainframe." Paul shook hands with Matthew and left him. Matthew watched Paul go to his car. He walked back to his desk, sat down, and began doodling concentric circles right next to a whole column of figures before it hit him. Matthew always thought he was fine. He was handling this Christiane thing OK. And then it would hit him. The quiet sobbing came first. And then, uncontrollable tears and dry heaves that racked his entire body. There was no solace, no relief. He managed to drag himself through most days by telling himself he was making sure there would be fewer Christianes. But no matter, even when he thought he had finally licked this thing. One minute he was fine, talking to Paul or whomever, and the next minute, his whole body emitted the total anguish that he had managed to repress for so many days, months, years.

*Christiane*

*Year 2055*

*Christiane worked with supreme concentration, head bent over the grass box as she tended her window garden. Her condo was special for the window boxes she had. Some, of course, were situated only at light boxes; she couldn't afford a place with too many windows. The unique color of the grass held her gaze and she breathed deeply. Some people didn't notice that grass had an odor, but Christiane did. She smiled. Maybe the perfect man for her would be someone with similar olfactory talents! She tossed her thick strawberry blonde hair back and breathed deeply. She sat back in her chair and turned her attention to the new computer program she had just downloaded. "All About 20th Century Gardens" contained the most amazing pictures. Historical really. She imagined rolling in so much grass. What would it feel like? Would it be cold or warm? If she had a garden, it would have to include a fountain and a circular path. Then flower beds. Flowers. She clicked onto that choice. Her hazel eyes clouded with the disappointment that her own boxes held only various types of grasses. Flowers would be a real luxury. Maybe in the future. Her dreamy eyes closed as she thought about Matthew. She knew he had a crush on her. Maybe he was the one. When he had approached her after accounting class and asked her to meet him for coffee, he had seemed nervous—a surprise since he was one of Professor Tuchman's favorite students. Matthew always scored highest on the exams and obviously stayed up to date on the latest laws coming over the internet. His self-assurance in class appealed to Christiane. Matthew Salmund. Maybe he was the one.*

*Christiane cleaned up the soil that had spilled onto the table where she had been working. She carefully laid her gardening tools in the drawer where they belonged; grabbed her bookbag and keys and headed out the door of her condo. When she reached the street she looked up at the sky. Remembering how the sky looked on the computer, she frowned. Once upon a time the sky was blue. The only sky she had ever seen was gray. Always gray. So boring. Never one to dwell on sad stuff, Christiane headed toward the University Coffee Shop and wondered what Matthew liked to do for fun.*

*Matthew arrived five minutes early and luckily found a table. The students crowded into the coffee shop at all hours. Matthew's priorities until now had not included girls. His goal was to make it through the grueling accounting courses at the Sylvia Gaupp University and graduate first in his class. Accounting jobs were sought after in these times, and Matthew did not want to be left out. He seldom took time for leisure activities, but something about Christiane had made him reassess his life. His parents both worked in the postal service and lived modestly. They did not really understand Matthew's drive to achieve. In fact, they openly worried about him. Matthew didn't know where it came from—this need to be constantly busy, always striving. He had arrived on campus, ready to work as hard as he could for the three year course of study in accounting. And now he was deviating from that path, he knew. Girlfriends could take up a lot of valuable study time. But he couldn't resist, he thought, as he took another look at the door watchfully waiting for her entrance. He scanned the room. Why was she different from all the others? He had never had any interest in friends or social activities. But there was something about Christiane. She made him feel excited in a way that was new to him. His gaze wandered over the room one more time and then back to the doorway.*

*And there she stood! Her eyes brightly searched and then came to rest on his. He smiled back and felt ridiculous. He wasn't supposed to care like this. No turning back now. She made her way through the maze of little round tables to him.*

*"Hello! You found us a table! And near the window too! I love windows!"*

*"I'm glad you approve. Please sit. What kind of coffee do you want?"*

*Christiane smiled. "Is it OK if I have tea? I'm really not a coffee drinker."*

*"Sure. I'll go put our order in. Be right back. Don't move."*

*"Oh, no! I wouldn't want to lose this spot." She smiled back, her eyes holding Matthew in a trance so that he bumped into another student as he headed toward counter service, but he couldn't let go of her gaze. Get a grip he told himself. This isn't healthy. The place was noisy but he knew, even though he was across the room, that she was giggling. She's laughing at me, and I like it. There is something very wrong with me. All I can think about is I want to touch her hair. It doesn't look like she even colors it. And her skin. So many colors all seem to contribute to a refreshingly healthy aura. I'm sunk. What do I say to her? Matthew started to sweat. I never sweat. What is this? He placed his order. And tried not to turn around.*

*Across the room, Christiane was admiring his brown corduroy jacket and tan pants. The way his shoulders looked so broad. His dark brown hair accentuated*

55

*his dark eyes, which fascinated her. What secrets were there behind those eyes? Could she get him to smile more?*

*As he headed back to their table carrying a tray with coffee and tea in hand, Matthew made a decision. He would not try to impress her. He would be just himself. He didn't want to get himself in too deep with this girl. And if he really just behaved his usual natural way, surely she would not be interested. His eyes on his tray, he didn't notice Christiane's playful smile. He's so serious, he's cute, she thought.*

*"You know, you're not like most of the guys I hang out with."*

*"Oh really, how am I different?"*

*"Well, for one thing, you're very serious. And a good student. And you carry coffee really well. In addition to which you don't make me go get my own. I think this is a first actually for me. You must spend a lot of time studying which, again, is totally different from the guys I'm usually with."*

*"I really don't work that hard."*

*"Oh, yes, you do. You always are one step ahead of Professor Tuckman. The rest of us are in awe. Really we are."*

*"You probably get good grades."*

*"Oh, I do alright," she smiled coyly. Christiane did a very good job of keeping her high IQ hidden from sight when she was with her friends. But somehow she didn't mind Matthew knowing. "I'm not really into accounting. I'm planning to go into law. My parents are both lawyers, and I guess it kind of rubbed off." She gave him a dazzling smile. "So, Matthew what do you like to do for fun?"*

*"Fun? Fun doesn't really exist for me, usually, that is. I mean this is fun right now. Being here with you, I mean." Oh no, was he stammering? And he felt so hot. "And I guess I have to admit having fun is the one thing I'm not really good at. You might find me actually kind of boring." Matthew looked into Christiane's large eyes that seemed to pull at him. I'm a goner he thought to himself. She's got me. How am I going to keep her?*

*Christiane felt her insides tugging. A new feeling. Guys were guys. You didn't have real conversations with them, did you? This guy was so honest. So sincere. Guys didn't do that. Could you really be close to a guy? The way you are close to your best girlfriend?*

*Time went by and Matthew worked at keeping the conversation going. He didn't want her thinking he couldn't even talk. Finally, he paused at which time Christiane said, "Maybe you're not so boring. Maybe you are more interesting than you think. You know I have to get going to my civil law class. This was really nice. I mean you did a good job with the tray and all." She laughed. "Maybe we could do this again?" She looked at him questioningly, eyebrows raised.*

*"Sure, sure. I'd like that! Maybe you can turn me into one of those fun guys you usually hang out with!"*

*She gave him one more smile before turning to leave. "Maybe I don't want to." She slung her bookbag over her shoulder and looked intently at him. "See you in class."*

*And she was gone. And all of the air and light went out of the room. The energy of her presence was not gone though and Matthew realized he wanted more of it. Suddenly life without the force of Christiane seemed dull. Even his goal of becoming a successful accountant seemed silly if life didn't include this zest named Christiane. Snap out of it, he told himself. This is crazy.*

*A week had passed since her "meeting" with Matthew. She couldn't really call it a date. And though she had seen Matthew several times since then, he or she had always been in a hurry. So maybe it was just a wrinkle in life. Like she had read about in one of her spiritual guides. She tried to restrain herself from thinking too much about things spiritual. After all, spirituality was really just a myth. Her parents had taught her to be rational, logical, cause and effect and all that. But there were these nagging phrases that she couldn't forget once she'd seen them on the internet. Whatever. She pushed it all out of her mind and turned her attention to her grass box. The grass had sprouted beautifully in her latest creation and actually needed a little trimming. A task she now occupied herself with while trying NOT to think about Matthew.*

*Yuck! She wrinkled her nose and took a sip of tea from the mug that said, "Let your spirit guide you" on her work table. She continued her internal dialogue, I mean I really want to be a lawyer eventually, but right now I don't know. I'm young, and I just want to have a good time. No emotional strings please. She stood up and took a look at herself in the full length mirror. "I don't want to care about Matthew," she said firmly and aloud to her reflection. And then she started laughing. "I'm a nut. Good thing I keep that hidden from everybody. And I must keep it from Matthew," she said in a deep voice. Hey girl, get back to the grass.*

*And then there was Paul. Paul had recently joined Christiane's Constitutional Law study group and seemed determined to be Christiane's friend. Which was OK. Because not only was Paul pretty smart, he turned out to be a lot of fun. They began frequenting the virtual games room at the College Student Union. Paul's gregarious behavior and relaxed manner made him easy to be around. Like today. Paul had caught Christiane staring at Matthew as they headed out of class together.*

*"Why are you mooning over that brain mass?"*

*"Oh I'm not!"*

*"Come on"*

*"All right! Maybe I do think he's cute. We had coffee, and he hasn't paid any attention since. So that's all there is to it."*

*Paul took another look in Matthew's direction. "He's a brain mass minus a few. Anyone would be crazy to fall for—I mean ignore you." Paul gave her his toothy grin. His grin and his freckles. That's what made Paul just a little bit different. His reddish hair, blue eyes and lanky build accentuated his quirky personality. He was passionate about law though. She had seen him in action at mock trials in class. When he was lawyering, he was a completely different person. His serious side emerged and woe to any opponent. Christiane had breathed a sigh of relief when her name had not been chosen to argue opposite him.*

*"I tell you what," Paul was saying. "I can help you out with this. Let's go get coffee and let's invite Matthew. Great idea, huh?"*

*So that was how they became a threesome. Three times a week and sometimes four, Paul, Matthew and Christiane met at the coffee shop. For the rest of the semester they talked about everything. They occasionally went to a movie or did a virtual thing together but most of the time it was just talk. Matthew and Christiane inched closer to one another. Paul just didn't get it. What was the holdup with these two? In the course of the spring semester, he had had already four different girlfriends and these two were still stumbling around each other. Oh well; they seemed happy enough. And life was so comfortable knowing the three had each other. They talked about everything. The latest games, politics, other students, their profs, and lately spirituality. Which was getting pretty weird. Christiane had recently admitted she logged on to spiritual pages pretty regularly. Matthew and Paul accepted this as just another Christiane Thing. She raised grass and she read about the spirits.*

*"Hey guys. I have a great idea. Let's go to the new greenhouse. It opens next week."*

*More grass! The three were at their usual table by the window having coffee and tea. Matthew and Paul looked at Christiane and then at each other as if they had rehearsed the scene.*

*Paul began, "What is with this girl?"*

*Matthew looked over at Christiane and spoke while looking intently into her eyes, "I don't know. But if we don't go, she'll never let it go. You know that." He didn't know it, but Christiane absolutely loved the way Matthew would look at her in that way that he had—as if she were all that existed. He could almost hypnotize her with his eyes.*

*Paul pretended not to notice. He always kept the repartee going even when Matt and Christiane had one of their moments. He chattered on. "It's true. How much is this going to cost. And can we wear disguises. Only weirdoes go to these places. Christiane, how far do we have to go to prove our love to you?"*

*Christiane snapped out of her reverie and looked at Paul indignantly. "Love! I thought you said love doesn't exist. That feelings like that are nonexistent. Life is just chemical reaction. How about that Paul. Huh?"*

*"I'm just trying to avoid one of our hour long discussions entitled the existence of . . . you fill in the blank, so we can get to class on time for a change." Christiane laughed good-naturedly and then stopped abruptly. Paul and Matthew both exchanged meaningful looks as Christiane's face tensed.*

*There was that twinge again. Ever so slight, so internal that Christiane wasn't sure she felt it. This morning she had spent extra time getting dressed, checking herself several times in the mirror. Was it her imagination or was her hair thinning, and what about her skin? It was taking more and more makeup to cover up the fact that her once golden flesh was turning gray—the color of the sky, she thought ruefully. Christiane had always taken pride in her healthful lifestyle. At age nineteen she certainly didn't expect to have to concern herself with health problems. Suddenly her body was not keeping up. Fatigue had become a frequent companion. And Matt and Paul were starting to notice. They hadn't said anything but she had caught both of them on separate occasions staring at her face with what looked like worry and even distaste.*

*Christiane summoned up all the strength she could and announced that she needed to stop at her condo before hustling off to class and assured Matt and Paul that she would meet them there.*

*They both turned to watch her leave. Then Paul said, "Well, Matt, what do you think?"*

*"She certainly seems concerned about something. I grant you that. What do you think is going on with her? She is not usually secretive. Do you think she has a boyfriend?"*

*Paul gave Matt a disgusted look and said sarcastically, "Yes, I know she has a boyfriend. I'm looking at him. It isn't that. You know it too. There's something going on. Maybe I'll stop in on her tonight since I'm NOT the boyfriend, and she might confide in me."*

*For the first time in her life, school had become a burden. This feeling surprised Christiane, always having been a person of great energy who prided herself on not getting sick. No longer could she pretend to herself. Something very wrong had taken over her body. She had ignored the discomfort and other physical changes long enough. The only course of action remaining was a visit to the doctor. She started by visiting the health office at school. Following Professor Tuckman's class, and after making up some lame excuse to Paul and Matt, she had walked purposefully over to the Marion Building which housed the student health office.*

*Once there, she signed in, gave her information and identification number to the receptionist, and sat down to wait. Christiane mentally listed her symptoms— tired all the time, losing weight without even trying, moments when she couldn't work with her garden tools. Maybe she was studying too hard she thought to herself. You're making too much of this. Oh well the doctor will tell me as much, and I'll go on my merry way.*

*"Christiane," a very nice young man had walked over to where she was sitting in the waiting room and asked her to follow him down the hall to exam room number five. He pointed to a gown lying on the exam table and left her there. Christiane closed the door, changed into the gown and sat up on the table. Just stay calm she told herself. It's really nothing. Presently a young girl entered the room. She looked young to be a doctor. Not much older than Christiane.*

*"Hi Christiane, my name is Karen. I'm your caregiver today. Could you explain why you are here?" Christiane began slowly to describe her various discomforts including how she had dragged herself here to the student health office today.*

*"Maybe I'm just working at my classes too hard," she said as she finished her recitation.*

*"That may be," Karen replied. "We are going to do some blood tests today, and I will do an EKG. It's probably nothing to worry about, Okay?"*

*Relieved just to have confided in someone, Christiane nodded and thanked Karen.*

*Once she had reached home, Christiane tossed off her shoes and climbed into bed under the deliciously warm blankets. Sleep came almost immediately, and she dreamed deeply of green fields and blue skies. Suddenly, she heard something like thunder and, startled, woke up to the knocking sound of her door. She took a minute to remember where and when, then headed to see who was at the door at seven o'clock at night. She checked the peephole and saw Paul on the other side. Christiane took a minute to look in the mirror and was aghast at what she saw. She only looked worse than ever. She grabbed a hairbrush and lipstick and did the best she could. Resignedly she opened the door.*

*"Hi Paul. What are you doing over in these parts tonight?"*

*"I came to see you, of course." Paul noticed that Christiane wouldn't look at him. It even seemed to him that she was trying to keep her back turned to him. "What is going on with you Christiane? Are you mad at me or Matt? Is something going on that you don't want to tell us? Did we do something we shouldn't? Are you sick of us hanging around? Come on, give, what is it?"*

*Christiane turned to face him. She watched the alarm on his face as he saw her now with minimal makeup. "Something is wrong with me. I don't know what. I went to student health today. They're doing some tests and will call me. It's probably nothing serious. Maybe I'm anemic. I know I look awful. And I wouldn't blame you or Matt if you didn't want to hang out with me. I could never be angry with you guys."*

*"Come on! You're my best buddy and I don't desert a friend and besides, you look great!" Paul put his arm around Chris and walked her over to the window. "You're a beautiful girl, Christiane, and if Matt hadn't latched on to you first, you know I'd be after you. In fact, aren't you done with him yet? He's boring— you know that, and I'm not. Don't tell him I said that, but you know it's true."*

*Christiane smiled, "You are right about one thing. I think I finally love someone—something besides my grass and sky computer programs. I thought it would never happen and I'll never know why it happened with Matt. And I'm very into him. But, just look at me!" Suddenly the tears came. She collapsed onto the sofa crying. "Why would he want to hang on to me?" Paul sat down next to her and held her for a very long time.*

*Later that evening, Paul met Matt for dinner.*

*"So what's the deal?" Matt asked. "You went to see her. You didn't try anything, did you?"*

*"Of course not! You know I would never move in on you and Chris. No, it was like I told you. I just went to see her to find out what was going on. She's not feeling well just like we thought. Thinks it is anemia. She is getting it checked out, so don't worry about it, and whatever you do, don't let her know how bad she looks. Just tell her how beautiful she is. When they figure this out, they'll put her on iron or whatever and she will be fine in no time and you'll be glad you stuck with her."*

*"You think I'd let her go just because of her looks?" Matthew paused, honestly, would he? He tried to imagine life without the one person who liked him, truly liked him in spite of his boring nature and discomfort around people. She really seemed to care about him. How could he possibly think he could do without her?*

*He looked at Paul "We'll be together forever. You'll see" and he was dead serious.*

*The alarm went off. Christiane opened her eyes and tried to discern her condition for the day. The pain in her back had worsened. She had absolutely no desire to get out of bed ever again. She didn't care about seeing anybody, even Matt or Paul. School was a distant memory even though she knew she had made it to two of her classes just yesterday. With great effort she rolled over to her side thinking she would make it out of bed, but found just that much effort exhausted her. Her eyes closed and she slept. The phone rang on her bedside table, and she reached for the receiver.*

*"Hello."*

*"Hello, Christiane? This is Karen from the health center. We got your results back, and they were inconclusive. Could you come back, so we can get you together with a PA?"*

*"Oh, I thought you were the PA?"*

*"Uh, no. Really, I'm just a tech."*

*"Oh. Hmmm. Sure, sure, when do you want me to come by?"*

*"Three o'clock tomorrow, OK with you? We're kind of busy today."*

*"Sure, I'll be there tomorrow three o'clock."*

*Chris dropped the receiver onto the cradle and slept again. Now the door. Wouldn't anyone let her rest? She dragged herself out of bed and limped with pain to the door. Matthew this time, she thought irritably. Slowly she pulled open the door and immediately headed to the couch to fall into a semi-reclined position. Alarmed, Matt hurried over to her and held her face in his hands.*

*"Christiane, what is going on here? You don't look well. What did the doctor say?"*

*"Oh, I'm going back for an appointment tomorrow. They'll figure it out I'm just really tired." She lied, of course. Her back was killing her, and the headache she started with yesterday was only getting worse.*

*Matt put his arms around her and felt her bony rib cage jutting out in a way that was new. "Aren't you eating?"*

*"Yeah, I ate just yesterday. I had some soup, I think."*

*"I'm taking you to the hospital right now. We're going to get to the bottom of this right now. You're sick and I can't stand to see you like this."*

*Matthew dialed 911 helpline on Christiane's computer. A form appeared. He typed in Christiane's name and address.*

*He ran over to the sofa where Christiane had collapsed and fallen asleep. He gently roused her. "What's your social security number?" She looked at him, blank for a minute then gave it to him.*

*Then the web site asked him to classify her illness, life-threatening emergency, severe emergency, emergency care may be needed, chronic problem never treated before or chronic problem, hospitalized before. Frantic, Matthew took another look at Chris across the room on the sofa. He'd heard of refusals to treat by hospitals if you exaggerated the level of care required. What did he know about all this? He was an accounting major for God's sake. He cursed himself for not going into the medical field. If he had, he could help the one person he loved right now. What would juggling numbers ever do for her? He thought about asking Chris. But another look her way told him she had dozed off. He'd have to risk his own judgment on this. He chose emergency care may be needed and hit send.*

*He looked at his watch. Two o'clock p.m. He went back over to Chris and sat. Time passed and he realized he should pack a suitcase for her in case they did admit her to the hospital. He took a quick look at her. She slept quietly. He headed into her bedroom. He rummaged through the closet and behind some old pillow, No, it was a stuffed animal toy, a bear, he thought. It was so worn he couldn't tell for sure. He pushed whatever it was aside and found a sports type satchel, which he dragged out and took over to her bureau. He checked his watch (thirty minutes had passed since he sent for the ambulance). He pulled some nightwear, underwear and socks out of the drawers. He checked the closet again and found a pair of slippers. He wanted her to be comfortable in the hospital. He planned to stay with her the whole time. He smiled briefly to himself as he realized that normally he never missed a class and now his schoolwork seemed to be completely out of his mind—another time and space that didn't exist for him at this moment. He had to get her well. His life had only meant something real to him since he had met her. He thought about how energetic he felt after being around her. He looked at his watch. Forty-five minutes. When were they coming?*

*He went back to check on Christiane, Her breathing appeared labored. He studied her thin, bony frame and realized how much she had changed physically since he had met her. How long had she been in pain and said nothing? Why hadn't she told him before? One hour. That was it. He went back to the screen and pulled up his 911 emergency request. He looked at the box he had checked next to May Be an Emergency. He moved the clicker over to it to erase and change to the highest level. The clicker did not respond, He tried a manual request. Nothing. Then after trying the clicker a number of times, a notice appeared on the screen. REQUEST HAS BEEN SENT AND MAY NOT BE CHANGED. Matt grabbed hold of the monitor and shook it.*

*"That won't change things." Christiane said quietly from her sofa. "Maybe you should drive me. I think I can walk."*

*"You know they won't admit you if you can walk in."*

*"That's OK. I don't want to stay there anyway. Come on; let's go."*

*Feeling defeated and at a loss, Matt walked over to her, put down the overnight bag he had packed, and reached down to carefully pick her up. She was so light.*

*"You don't have to carry me," she said embarrassed at having to be helped in such a way. "I can walk, really." But she allowed him to pick her up anyway; she felt so tired.*

*"You're fine. Everything about you is fine. Except this sickness thing. We've got to solve it Christiane. We've got to get you well. I'm a selfish person and I need you well."*

*She smiled. "Together we can do it. I know it." They were both pretending to be optimistic, he knew, as he reached down to pick up her overnight bag while still carrying her.*

*The PA who eventually saw them (a three hour wait wasn't bad, they said) was really very nice and concerned. Unfortunately, Matt had the clear impression that this particular PA had no idea what the problem was with Christiane. He did give her iron pills and seemed unconcerned. When they left and Matt took Christiane back home, she did seem to have a bit of her old spark. She even suggested they cook something. Matt insisted she sit down while he set to the task of making an omelet for both of them.*

*"I don't like onions," she said when she told him she didn't have any.*

*With a show of exasperation, Matt took another look into her refrigerator and came up with scallions (She liked them because they looked like grass) and tomatoes. He chopped them both expertly.*

*"I'm so impressed," she said with her best pseudo deep voice accentuated by her fluttering eyelashes. He looked at her and smiled breathing inside a sigh of relief. She was going to be better. She just needed some rest and vitamins like the PA at the Wellness Center said.*

*A week passed and Matthew knew they both had to face reality. How could she have possibly lost more weight? She actually looked thinner that Friday night when he came over with the vegetarian Chinese food she had thought she could keep down. She was on the sofa as usual. "I live on this sofa," she thought ruefully as she waited for Matthew to arrive. He had said Paul might come over too. It would be like old times at the coffee shop. She stopped to think. How long had it been. Let's see. She never did take her midterms so it had been just about three months. Living on the sofa watching each day tick by. Paul had been really sweet and had brought her the latest books on spirituality. Some of them were hard to understand but others had words in them that brought her some sense of peace.*

*Matt remembered that night. When he saw the books Paul had brought, he wished he believed in God. He wished he could pray. He just didn't know how. And he didn't know of any other way to save Christiane. He knew that something was very wrong inside Christiane. He knew the end was coming. He knew they would try all sorts of things or maybe they wouldn't. With modern healthcare you never could tell which diseases they would treat and which they wouldn't. Political considerations took precedence over the health of the patient. Paul was thinking of going on to graduate school and doing research on it. Matt thought Paul was the lucky one—to be able to think of the future with some purpose in mind. He, Matt, could not look at a future without Christiane in it. He simply had no purpose except for her.*

*"Hey Beautiful!" Paul sang out that Friday night as Matt and he entered the room. The men had agreed that they would always talk about how beautiful Christiane was when they were with her. This was their gift to her. They pretended all was well. Even though that Friday night all three knew things were very wrong.*

*The two men ate heartily even though neither felt much like eating. They had decided that if they ate with her, maybe Christiane would eat more and gain some strength and weight back. And she did make a valiant effort every time. But it was a delicate balance between eating just enough that you could stand the nausea and eating too much so that you had to run to the bathroom to throw up. As a result, she was always even more exhausted when the two left her. The tension of pretending to be well, trying desperately not to throw up and keeping the mood light, as if she believed she was going to make it, took every last ounce of energy she had. After they left, she always slept soundly. Sometimes, Matt would stay and watch her sleep and dose, himself, through the night. She loved waking up and seeing him there in his unstylish, often wrinkled clothes, so he looked even more a mess.*

*The morning after the Chinese food, she awoke and saw Matt just in such a position. Suddenly, his eyes opened and he looked at her.*

*She smiled and asked, "Matt do you believe there is a higher power out there?" She saw that Matt looked a bit uncomfortable as he did whenever they talked about such things. Paul was much easier about it for some reason. "What I really mean is," and she whispered these words, "Is there more to life than what is here as we know it?" A tear formed in her right eye, but she kept looking at him. She had to ask. "Will I totally cease to exist when I die?" She knew she was being hard on him, but she had to know. Miraculously, Matt answered, "You will never cease to be you. There's got to be something out there. I know it. Don't forget that." She lay back down and rested her eyes and a smile formed on her lips. And now her tears ran freely.*

In his sumptuous office at Universal Health Club, Matt smiled now as he remembered how he lied about all that to Chris. He didn't regret it, only wished he truly believed it. When he had looked into those eyes that still held light, he knew she had wanted his reassurance. He had to give it to her. There was nothing else he could have done for her. As always he tortured himself with the memory of his inability to help—his own immaturity and lack of ability. If only were the two words that plagued him. If only was followed by such a long list of fill in the blanks that he could barely remember them all. But unfortunately he did all too well. If only ... always check the worst case box, be more pushy when someone tells you the simple answer that you know can't possibly be true (he wanted to believe so badly that it was just an iron problem). Pay more attention to the people who really matter—now that was a big one. And so quickly forgotten, but, like his other "if onlys," it popped up to greet him whenever he remembered the unique relationship he had with Christiane. Listen when your friends try to help you. Paul saw the change in Chris even before he did. Why didn't he listen? Be persistent. Why didn't they go back to the hospital the very next day when Chris' ribs made an odd sound and she felt pain different from any other. If only the first PA had admitted his lack of knowledge and called in someone else. That was the if only Matt worked on every day of his life. He owed it to Christiane. His love. The young girl at nineteen who didn't have to die. He dreamed about her so often that he had decided this was his punishment—not the dreams but waking up from the dream to know that he had failed her and he owed her big time. So this was how he had become a drug smuggler for the Underground. Every time he helped make a delivery, waking up was a little easier. He forced himself to remember now back to the day after the Chinese dinner.

*Paul and Matt decided to call the ambulance and use the top rating. The ambulance arrived in fifteen minutes and took Christiane to the Wellness Center. This time there was quite a fuss over her. A PA saw her and then a doctor. Soon a specialist arrived and that's when Christiane, Matt and Paul looked at each other and silently agreed they all knew how bad this was. The specialist worked on Christiane's case for the allotted three days and came up with the word Leukemia. A really aggressive Leukemia. Paul wondered wasn't it there before? Three months ago? A year ago? How had this been missed?*

*"Why can't she have the medicine?" Matt tried to be calm, reasonable. The doctor tried to explain once again.*

*"It's not available for cases like that of your friend." Matt noticed the doctor would not make eye contact.*

*"Look, you know it's what she needs. She's gotta have something. Can't you see the pain she's in? She's only nineteen. She can't possibly have used her allotment."*

*The doctor looked down at his feet and then nervously at his watch. "No, she hasn't, but she's too far advanced with this disease. Medicine won't stop it now."*

*"How do you know?" Matt noticed his own hands and knees were starting to shake. Anger surged through him. "HOW CAN YOU POSSIBLY KNOW IF SHE WILL MAKE IT?"*

*"Try to calm down. We know that she has only a twenty percent chance of recovery. All the studies show this. I'll lose my job if I go ahead with this. You've got to be reasonable about this."*

*"YOU'LL LOSE YOUR JOB?! SHE'S GOING TO LOSE HER LIFE AND YOU KNOW IT. WHAT KIND OF A DOCTOR ARE YOU?"*

*"Look, it's hard to accept, I know."*

*"YOU DON'T KNOW!" Matt slammed the door as he left. Where to go now? What to do? He stood leaning against the wall outside the doctor's office and tried to calm down. Sweat poured down from the temple of his forehead. Paul found him a few minutes later.*

*"Come on, let's get some coffee. There's got to be another way." Matt spent the next twenty minutes bringing Paul up to speed on what had happened between the doctor and him.*

*"I can't go in to see her knowing this, Paul. I can't tell her they've given up on her. The medicine could work, but the lousy government goes with the odds. Betting on Chris' life. It's sick."*

*"Matt, hear me out. There may be another way. I've been doing some interning at the Star Line News Organization. You know, nothing really important—just junk work that they need done, and they don't have to pay me since I'm a student and all. But here's the thing, and I've been thinking about this for a long time. I don't want to get anybody in trouble especially not you and not Chris. But sometimes I do some computer input for the health section and while I'm sitting there, I'm sort of invisible to everyone who comes into the editor's office. They—you know—editors from all over—they talk to each other. They all have code names and they email all day long about all sorts of stuff. Stuff they can't put out for the public. Stuff that they know about, but don't put in the news. That's why I want to get into the news reporting business more than ever. The knowledge—the real knowledge about how the government really works—not just the web page version. Anyway, there's a drug Underground."*

*"That's your big news?" Matt said bitterly. "That's been around since forever. You're kidding, right?"*

*"No listen, I'm not talking uppers and downers and mood changers. I'm talking drugs that are legitimately used for health reasons. Remember when pot was illegal but still cancer sufferers used it. People who weren't criminals. It's sort*

*of like that. You see. With all the restrictions the government has placed, the limitations and so on, well, there's a network, an illegal network but not necessarily bad or evil—you know a group of people who steal drugs that are legitimately needed but maybe the recipient's quota is filled or the family allotment is gone. Like that. So there's an Underground." Paul became more excited as he continued. "People who think anybody should be able to get any drug they need— for an illness—that is. It's dangerous. Maybe I shouldn't even suggest it. But members of Congress and other government agencies apparently use it all the time for their own healthcare. And the government just looks the other way for them. Of course, they're not gonna look the other way for us. We could go to jail. What? What …?"*

*Matt was beaming at him. "It's definitely worth it," he said eagerly. "But just Chris and me. You won't be involved. Just get us the info and then after that, you drop out of the whole thing. You don't know us. It's her only shot. I know it's the right thing. Let's do it. How can we find a contact? How do we get hooked up to this?"*

*"Matt, think about this. It could affect your whole future. And Chris may not make it anyway. Let's think about it for a day. One day couldn't make that much difference. Anyway, it'll take me that long to figure a way to get the information. How we're going to get the stuff. And it will probably cost us. I don't know how much. We can pool our money and see what we can do. But think. Just for a day. I'll come by your place tomorrow. No email chatting, no phones, OK?"*

*"I'm going to go talk to Chris."*

*"Hold off," Paul warned. "Don't get her hopes up. Matt, promise. I know you're excited. But promise. Okay?"*

*"Yeah, you're right. I'll just, I don't know, I'll tell her the doctor hasn't decided which medicine to use yet. That'll hold her for one day anyway."*

*The information highway had become Paul's life blood. Knowledge excited him like nothing else could. And hacking into computers had been a special skill of his ever since grade school. He didn't do it much anymore. He hadn't known there was any information that was not just yours for the taking. But in the last week sitting in the editor's office, cleaning up his files, he had learned more than a room full of computers could have taught him. How did the Underground keep track of its drugs? It was hard for him to believe they didn't have it on a disk somewhere. How could they communicate if not with the computer? More difficult than hacking into computers, Paul thought, would be getting the information he needed for Chris out of a person. Which person at the paper should he approach? Which one would be discreet? Who knew and would be gutsy enough to share that information with a college student like himself? His mind sifted through all the people he had met in the health department of the paper. And which ones had been in the office when the editor had been discussing the latest high-ranking official who had received medicines beyond the prescribed allotment.*

*There had been that weasel he couldn't stand, Henry something. And the secretary who really had just listened. The traveling reporter who seemed pretty knowledgeable about diseases and their treatments was a possibility. Marcie was her name. She was young, but seemed kind of distant. He felt uneasy about asking her. The editor, Jamy Savage, seemed pretty sharp. And Jamy seemed to like Paul, had even referred to him as a surrogate son, since Jamy had never had children. Career was everything to her. Paul had felt comfortable with her from the start. She said clearly what she meant and he knew she had that inborn rebellious streak that was so necessary in the information business world. He waited until they were alone. He had been working on Jamy's files for about an hour. She had just hung up from a transatlantic call.*

*Paul got up from his desk, walked over and stood in front of her. Jamy looked up and smiled. Paul was a favorite, even when compared to the many before him whose careers she had helped launch.*

*"What can I do for you Paul?"*

*Paul chose his words carefully. "I'd like to ask you for some information."*

*"Sure."*

*"Well this might be a little sensitive. You might not trust me with it. I want to assure you that I'm not some sort of spy or anything. I'm just a person who wants to help another person. And I think you might be able to help me."*

*"Sure, sure go ahead, Paul, you know I trust you. You're special to me. I like having you around and I think you have a great future in this business. Now go ahead, ask away."*

*"I have a friend. A really sick friend."*

*Jamy became concerned. "You don't mean yourself, do you? You're not hiding something from me, are you?"*

*"No! No, really. This friend. She has Leukemia."*

*"The thing is, they won't give my friend the medicine that will cure it."*

*"Well, Paul, there is probably a reason for that," Jamy replied reasonably.*

*"They told us she doesn't have a high enough percentage chance of recovery. They won't waste it on her."*

*Jamy noticed how suddenly Paul looked like a person much older than he really was. It was early for him to have to face such a reality.*

*"Sometimes, Paul, we have to accept things. Our system of healthcare is still the best in the world."*

*"I've heard you say just the opposite right here in this room," Paul blurted out loudly. That wasn't how he'd meant to proceed at all. He took a deep breath and thought for a minute. He noticed how carefully Jamy had all the little knick*

69

*knacks arranged on her steel desk. He looked into her face. She was watching him. And now he saw she had made a decision not to confide in him.*

*"I'm trustworthy," he pleaded.*

*There was a brisk knock on the door and Jamy yelled, "Come in." It was Marcie. She glanced from Paul to Jamy and back to Paul.*

*"I'll come back later."*

*"No, Marcie it's OK. Come on in. Paul and I are finished with what we were doing. Paul you can finish the files now if you want."*

*"No thanks. I've got a class. If it's all the same to you, I'll be back tomorrow." Paul answered bitterly. He looked from one to the other and left.*

*Matt wasn't going to like this at all. Paul felt like such a failure. Why wouldn't Jamy help him?*

*"What did he want?" Marcie asked Jamy.*

*"I think he wants in on the Underground. What do you think? Word is getting out somehow. How are we going to help everyone? How are we going to decide? Are we going to become like the government system by limiting access?"*

*"Let's just worry about Paul and his friend right now. You know we are on the right side on this. We will do the most that we can. Look I'll have to do a check on him and his family before anyone will be willing to trust him. You know the routine."*

*"I know but it was so hard to refuse him. He appears desperate. I hope he doesn't do anything stupid."*

*"I'll work as fast as I can on this one. You keep your profile low as usual. Maybe think about a way to give Paul a future in editorial reporting?" Marcie looked at Jamy meaningfully.*

*Sleep was out of the question for Paul that night. He had had a disappointing phone conversation with Matt in which he learned that Chris was now in the Wellness Center's Recovery Center. In Chris' case, this just meant that either she would recover or she wouldn't. Matt was totally out of it on the phone, barely able to spit out sentences, and totally without any hope.*

*The first call came at eight o'clock in the morning. Christiane had died. Marcie's call (unfortunately for her) came through at nine o'clock.*

*"I've got great news for you and your friend." Marcie started cheerfully.*

*"Oh really?"*

*"Yeah! I want to come over and see you. Is now convenient?"*

*"Yeah, sure." It was real convenient. He had forever. Paul had forever. And Chris was gone. The first call had been Matt. "She was in my arms one minute sleeping, smiling when she wasn't wincing from the pain, and then nothing."*

*By the time Marcie arrived at Paul's apartment, Matt was there also. The two sat in the living room not crying anymore. Just sitting, staring vacantly. Paul answered the door when Marcie rang. Paul looked awful as did his friend. Two lost young men. Totally dejected. Marcie stayed for just a short time. She had already learned to keep a distance from any of the clients she helped.*

So began the resolve of Matthew and Paul—the guilt so great, the desire to help so strong and the total inability to do anything to help a person who needed that help combined to create two very determined young men. Years passed. They both succeeded in their careers, but they both knew their real job of helping people in a way they had not helped Chris came first and foremost in their lives. No family for either one. The Underground came first.

# CHAPTER 12

## Year 2075

Baltimore City Police Department Precinct 23 was bustling with activity this Monday morning. Rufuos headed directly to the kitchen to make coffee. He'd had a great weekend with Stacey and the kids. Last night the youngest, Ginny had them up with a cough. Wore everybody out. That went along with having kids, and Rufuos didn't mind too much. He relished his role as a father and liked his work as a cop. But still Monday always rolled around too quickly. He poured the coffee into the coffee maker and returned to his desk to take a quick look at the morning news page on his computer while the coffee brewed. Not much of note happening. Boring is good he thought. The smell of freshly brewed coffee soon filled the air and Rufuos headed back to the kitchen, found his mug in the cupboard, poured his coffee and headed back to his desk, hoping for a quiet morning. Sis walked by just as he sat down. His quick glance noted the dark circles under her usually bright blue eyes. Mondays. So hard to get back into the swing of things he thought. Hopefully, the criminals would lay quiet today. Give him a chance to ease himself to work. The phone rang. No such luck.

"Hello, King here, 23rd precinct." he answered.

"Hey, Rufuos, it's just Hank downstairs at the front desk. There's a lady by the name of Gail Tilden here. I think you're the one she wants to talk to. Remember that missing person's report that you were interested in? The guy worked at Wellness? This is his wife down here. Wants to talk to you. Should I send her on up?"

"Yeah, send her on up," Rufuos said. "Guess the week's gotta begin sometime."

"OK, will do, and I'll try to spread the fun around!"

"Yeah, you do that, Hank. Do me a favor. Don't think of me next time or for the rest of the week for that matter. I'm having enough fun." Rufuos chuckled and hung up the phone. He grabbed his pad and paper, looked around for Sis wondering if she wanted in on this case and headed to the door to greet Ms. Tilden.

Making assessments about people and making decisions on how to solve problems were the two qualities Rufuos thought most important in cops. He felt pretty confident about his ability level in both areas. He thought about this now as he listened to Ms. Gail Tilden describe the disappearance of her husband, oddly, in a most detached way.

"He just didn't come home from work last Thursday. I thought he might have just decided, you know, to take a little break from things. I know before I met him, he sometimes would go off for a day or so, particularly if he was bothered by something at work. Anyway, I don't know where he's gone. For some reason the officer I spoke to Friday seemed to think he'd gone underground. The man at the front desk seemed to think you would know something about this, that you've been investigating the health clubs in the area for a possible connection."

"Connection?"

"To the Underground. You know, Underground hospitals and medical services."

"Well, it is true that we are interested in the Underground, of course, along with the Black Market, but I've come up with nothing about your husband. What's his name again?"

"Macklin. John Macklin. He's been a caregiver at the Wellness Center for three years now. They said he didn't turn in his bracelet. I really don't think he would involve himself with the Black Market, but the Underground? Yes, I can see him getting involved with that. Maybe you have an idea where he went?"

"I really don't," Rufuos studied her. She was young, pretty, with stylishly streaked hair, extremely well dressed. Untouched by life. A little uppity he thought, just a touch condescending. But she was government. Hell, so was he, but somehow they were so different.

She fidgeted a bit in her chair and then said, "I've talked things over with my boss, and we both agreed that I should go undercover."

Rufuos almost groaned aloud, caught himself just in time, and said as politely as possible, "I'm sure you're quite talented, but I've got a partner." He noticed Sis watching with a barely perceptible smile. "We're used to each other. I don't think I could really handle another." Rufuos glanced over at Sis.

"Oh, no! I didn't mean that," she answered. "I just want a way in."

"In?"

"Yes! In. Into the Underground. They already have plenty of agents infiltrating the Black Market. The government in the past has focused all of its resources on the Black Market. We know there is also a second underground organization that provides healthcare free." She paused. "I don't think my husband would have the chutzpah for anything so dangerous as the Black Market, but I can see him going to the Underground. And if I could go undercover in that organization, I might learn more and might even find my husband. I just came to you for a way in. I was told that you might know who could get me in. For a price, of course. The government is aware of how things are done on the outside."

Rufuos tried not to let the relief show on his face. He was a terrible poker player. "Let me think on that a minute." He mused for a moment, then reached into his file drawer and pulled his notes from last week. He studied Ms. Tilden's well thought out black and red suit accessorized with just the right bracelet and scarf. He looked at his list of names. And, God forgive him, Chuck Waller's just jumped right out of the page. The perfect match. The degenerate would be just right for Ms. Tilden's beginning of life education at Rufuos King's college. He pulled a photo of Mr. Waller out of the file and handed it proudly over to Ms. Tilden.

"Here you go. The perfect contact. He procures drugs for the Underground. He'll be able to get you in. And I don't think he'll even charge too much."

Ms. Tilden's carefully made up eyes brightened. She smiled and thanked Rufuos. Conspiratorially, she leaned down to his ear and told him she would be happy to share information. Oh please, Rufuos thought.

Oh gross, Sis thought as she watched with a grin from her desk.

"What was all that about?" Sis said when she saw that Ms. Tilden had made it out the door.

"Oh, that's one of those Medical Reports Agents—wants to find the Underground—wanted a contact."

"Rufe, you did warn her to stay away from the Black Market, didn't you? You did tell her just how dangerous they are, right?"

"She already seemed to know."

"Seemed to know? She didn't look like she knew anything about anything!"

Rufuos shrugged sheepishly, "Sis, I can't hold everybody's hand. I gave her Waller. We'll let him explain it to her." He turned to look at Sis. Their eyes met. "Want to go watch?" In unison they grabbed their notepads and caps and raced down to their car. The week was on.

Gail Tilden had led heretofore an orderly life: the right high school, college, an excellent score on the civil service test, a coveted job in the government, a decent looking husband who, up until now, had given her everything she wanted in a husband. What was with him anyway?

Infiltrating the Underground had not been totally her idea. Her supervisor was pushing for more information from Gail. And up until now, Gail really hadn't made any great finds. Gail worried that she would never be promoted. She didn't want to have to admit to her friends that she had the same dead end job she had gotten just out of college. So when John disappeared, Gail, having become immediately suspicious that he had gone under, began to think about following him—seemingly to find him but there *was* that job promotion she would like. And a new apartment would be REALLY nice. Having John back would be good, but she could always do an online divorce since they didn't have kids. So really, no biggie there. It would be obnoxious having to admit to her parents what had happened, but a superlative report from her supervisor regarding the Underground would help them forget all about her silly marriage to John. Just a childhood fling. Now she was taking responsibility, heading for a better job.

She drove down St. Paul Street away from the 23rd precinct and headed for the waterfront where she was supposed to be able to find this Waller character. If that smirking woman detective could do this sort of stuff, so could she. She was smarter, wasn't she? Had a college degree and all.

She found a place for her smart little car. Parked it and headed on foot to the water's edge. Checking the street signs she found the corner where this Waller guy was due. She took another look at the

picture Officer King had given her. He was certainly a decrepit looking character. Any place else he would stand out, but down here on
the waterfront, she was the one getting the stares. All sorts of shady
looking creatures passed her by and stared at her up and down. It was
all starting to make her very uncomfortable, when along came a guy
who looked familiar. It was him! Chuck Waller in the flesh, and, boy,
was there a lot of it. As he approached, she nervously fingered the
envelope full of cash that had been issued to her this morning. He
almost had passed her when she found the courage to reach out and
touch his arm.

"Mr. Waller?"

Chuck Waller had been busy deciding where lunch was coming
from today when this uptight but very good looking girl stopped him.
Things were looking up for good ole Chuck.

"Hey there, babe, what can I do for you?"

"Are you Chuck Waller?"

"Standing before you. At your service." He did his best to appear
noble in the presence of someone who obviously didn't frequent this
area.

"Could I have a moment of your time?" She knew she was supposed to identify herself as a government employee, but she had
already decided she didn't like this guy and certainly didn't trust him.
That officer had to have known this wasn't the kind of person she
wanted to be hooked up with.

"Sure babe, got lots of that. What can I do for you?"

Gail struggled to maintain her composure while trying not to let
the smell of liquor emanating from Mr. Waller's breath get the better
of her. She began to overheat. The stylishly cut blue wool coat she
was wearing weighed on her.

"I'd like to buy something from you," she managed. "Um, some
information, you might say."

Warning bells went off inside Waller's brain. His visceral survival
instinct heightened all of his senses. He started to back away.

"I have money," she blurted out. "Lots of money." She saw him
change, become interested. "I need to get into the Underground. I
need help getting into the Underground." She tried to hide the desperation in her voice.

"Why? Are you an agent?"

"They have my husband," she ignored his question. "I mean my
husband ran off with some of them. I just need someone, you know,

76

like you to vouch for me, to say I'm OK. To let me in. I could help. I know it. I could be of use. I know some pretty important people."

"Why should I help you? I don't even know you. How'd you find me? Where'd you get the money?"

Gail had her hand on the envelope filled with money.

Waller had his on a knife. So much better than guns in his opinion. So quiet. And here, by the water, she would be gone in no time. The current would take her body right outta here.

Giving up, Gail began to move away from this Chuck Waller. She backed away and then started off at a hurried pace heading directly for the street where the most people were.

"Hey wait. Ya didn't give me a chance. How much money?"

Gail turned swiftly, "Oh lots."

"OK, wait up. Let me see it."

"You must be kidding!"

"Well, how much?"

"Too much for the likes of you. You don't want to help. Fine. I'll find someone who will. I'm going to find my husband," she said determinedly.

What a rush! Gail sat down on the city bench right in the middle of Baltimore City Plaza and laughed out loud. What a rush! She had never felt this kind of excitement before. She couldn't believe what she had just done. And, she thought wickedly, she had kept half of the money for future expenses. That slob had been happy with the half. She had gotten not only a name but a place out of him. She had never realized how boring her life had been up until now. This was so different from anything in her life. Her conventional, predictable life. She had convinced a lowlife, streetwise bum like Waller to give her info, and she had done it without revealing her real name or true occupation. Some inner resolve had carried her—some sort of strength she didn't even know she had, had guided her. Turning away and leaving when she had no other leads but him—what had made her do that? All of her impulses had been the right ones. It all had worked out so perfectly. Plus, she had money to pay off the next person she came up against in this little adventure of hers. She thought of John. He never would have been able to do what she just did. He really was sort of a wimp, she thought meanly.

He did run off from his job. I guess that took some decision making, she thought. She headed up Charles Street in search of the

Universal Health Club. Waller had described Matt Salmund as too good for his expensive suits. At least he wouldn't be a slob like Waller.

# CHAPTER 13

"I guess coffee breaks don't happen here?" He had been at St. Luke's Hospital two days now, and, between not getting his usual meds and working non stop, John Macklin began to wonder about his decision to stay. His inner self watched as he expertly inserted the IV into the patient's arm.

"I'm impressed," Chambers said.

Me too, thought John. If Chambers only knew just how John's inner self struggled to allow him to work competently without the usual support of drugs.

"Are you sure you are just a tech?" Chambers asked.

"Yep, all I ever did in the hospital."

"Do you want to learn more?" He had groaned inwardly when Reverend McClaren had assigned Macklin to him, but John's personality had emerged, and it turned out that he showed a real interest in the patient's care, and even listened attentively when Chambers explained the reasoning behind the care decisions being made for each patient.

McClaren smiled as he stood outside the room listening. For his part, he had not meant to punish Dr. Chambers by linking Macklin with him. On the contrary, he liked Chambers. He liked him very much, but he worried that Chambers' intensity would burn him up. Chambers had amazing diagnostic abilities when it came to medical matters, but bedside manner—just too serious. McClaren believed Chambers needed to hold on to the intensity while at least appearing more relaxed when talking to the patients.

Maybe St. Luke's was the place. Maybe that's why Chambers had come to him. He had paired Macklin with him thinking that perhaps Macklin was the answer as well. They had found him on the roadside. How appropriate, McClaren thought. People made fun of him and his beliefs, he knew, but they couldn't make his faith waiver. The medical world both above and below ground discounted any sense of God. He knew that, but still he provided a haven that he knew they used without being part of his congregation. He knew, but still he hoped. Hoped that people like Marilyn, scientists, would someday have a place for religion in their scientific world. He prayed for every patient who came through St. Luke's. He prayed for the doctors, nurses, techs, everyone. McClaren considered every aspect of the healing process important. McClaren had heard Macklin ask for coffee. He smiled again and headed for his study. Let nature take its course, he thought.

"Come on! Coffee! Have mercy on me!" Macklin cried again.

"We've only been working four hours. What did they teach you at that government playground where you worked?"

"Oh, yeah, dump on me again. You're just too good for me. I know it. Sometimes I wonder why you and that Marcie chick picked me up."

Stephen looked at him, "Could it be you appeared rather desperate?"

"I guess I was." John admitted. He involuntarily rubbed his wrist, which did not go unnoticed by Chambers.

"So tell me, what was it like working at the Wellness Center?"

"It was OK. Boring. I didn't get to do half the stuff I do here. In fact, when I really look back on it, it was really pretty awful, monotonous. But I guess I needed that at the time. I didn't always work there. I had been in a pediatric intensive care unit before. I have to admit I couldn't handle it. I couldn't stand watching those little kids die. They got me into therapy, gave me some meds, pulled me out of there and put me in geriatric at Wellness. I guess they thought there was no suffering there, and sometimes that was true, but other times … Just because they're old, doesn't mean they don't suffer, you know? It was all so antiseptic, so sterile, nobody to talk to about the patients like you do here. Just give them what the computer says, and you're done."

"Then go have coffee," Chambers observed.

"Yeah, I guess that was it," John sheepishly admitted. "It was easy. As long as I didn't look into the patients' eyes, I was OK. I've watched you here. You seem detached, too, but you do think about the patients. Do you ever use the computer to check your diagnosis?"

"Actually, sometimes I do—just to check myself and also to see if there's another idea out there. Actually, *they* should be checking *our* computers. The government has suppressed many of the medical therapies that were commonly used—just to save money. What I am afraid of is losing all that information, information that it took researchers years to acquire. I'm afraid it will be no longer available to anyone. That's why the Underground is so important. Not only to deliver care, but to make sure that medical information makes it to the next generation of doctors. We need all the information, access to all studies done, even the ones that involve treatments and medicines the government does not want to pay for. Plus, I believe like my parents and grandfather, that patients need a human doctor with reasoning and problem solving abilities. The human body is too unpredictable and too variable. Of course, any studies supporting the use of human judgment versus computer decisions have been excised from the government computer libraries. The government also has deleted any studies that bear results they don't like. But even so, I check their computers. I want to be thorough, but it isn't likely I am going to find anything helpful there." He paused. "Hope I didn't bore you with all that."

"No. Scared me, yes. Bored me, no."

"Come on, let's go get that coffee."

There wasn't really a coffee room at St. Luke's Hospital, but there was a coffeemaker and a couple of chairs at the end of one of the wards. So John and Stephen sat there for a while drinking their coffee.

"I don't know about religion," Chambers began after they had both filled their mugs with coffee and sat down. "I don't think about it much. My parents were agnostics. I guess I'd say I'm an atheist. Guess I am what the government wants in that regard. How about you?"

"I never thought about it—not until recently when I had this old lady patient, Janis. She's the one I left for. She wanted to pray with me, I think. I couldn't even do that. I couldn't help her at all. When I look at what happened, I realize she helped me to see I needed to get out of there. That life didn't have to be that way. I never really had much of my own thoughts. I mean school told me what kind of job to get. Gail, that's my wife, she decided when I should get married, where I should work, what medicines even. Our apartment—all her idea—the way it's decorated, what we did every weekend, it was all her. Anyway, it got me thinking, this Janis' idea of praying—why couldn't I if I wanted to? Why couldn't I decide for myself? Why not stay with a patient a little longer if I thought it would help? Why always the stupid computer deciding how everyone in that hospital should function? So I just snapped, got out, left, left everything, even Gail. I bet she was surprised, shocked probably. She kind of looked down on me, probably already pushed the divorce through and told her friends some lie about what happened to me—something socially acceptable, like," he paused for emphasis, "I'm dead."

Macklin looked uncomfortable, so Chambers changed the subject. "We've got a new tech arriving soon—I think she is going to be working with computers, encrypting for us. McClaren's going to check her out and then we can meet her. Maybe she'll have some interesting news for us from the city. It can get boring here, too, I've discovered. It's good to have someone to talk to. Let's try to finish our rounds before the newcomer arrives."

John was pleased. Someone actually liked talking to him. "OK by me." John took Chambers' mug and returned them both to the cupboard after rinsing them.

# Chapter 14

McClaren saw Gail's car coming up the long driveway to St. Luke's. Their usual excitement and anticipation prevailed as the news of someone arriving from the city spread through the St. Luke's community. Everyone looked forward to news from the outside world. Though most didn't want to go back, he was sure there were some who missed it. He knew he did, but his life meant something here. It meant nothing in the city. Sunday service would be a quiet affair, always was, but he still worked on his message just as if he had hundreds of people listening. Wasn't one person just as important as the other ninety-nine in a hundred?

Here she comes now. Hopefully, the answer to their computer problems. Gail Tilden made a pretty picture coming up the steps to meet McClaren on the porch. Her perfectly cut shiny brown hair bounced as she walked.

"Ms. Tilden! Welcome. I'm Reverend McClaren. Hope your trip was satisfactory?"

"How do you do, Reverend. Thank you. Everything went well. No problem finding you." Gail looked around the dusty yard and turned to look into McClaren's eyes. "You're studying me aren't you?" she asked.

"I like to get to know my new people fast as I can," he responded.

"Well, I'm just an ordinary girl."

"I doubt that. First of all, nobody is ordinary in my book."

"And what book would that be, Reverend? The Bible?"

"Well, yes, I believe so," the minister answered thoughtfully. "Everyone is important. You know, a part of the whole, no job too small or unimportant. That's why we need you, Ms. Tilden. We need to communicate with other sites without worrying the wrong people might be listening in, you know?"

"I understand perfectly, and I'm sure I can help you."

"Do you know what we do here, Ms. Tilden?"

"I have some idea, I think."

"We're here to help people. That's about the size of it. Help them. We break some rules doing it. You know about rules, I'm sure. We, many of us, tried to live within the rules, but it just kept getting harder and harder 'til finally someone said, 'I can't do this anymore.' Got to make my own rules with God, you know, Ms. Tilden?"

At the mention of God's name, Gail became uncomfortable. Could she swing this? She didn't know. She had had some computer training in college and even encrypting class. She thought she could fake that part but she didn't know about this God stuff. She decided to play it straight. "Do I have to be into all that God stuff in order to help you?" she asked tentatively.

"No, of course not." McClaren laughed heartily. "You think these medical people here believe me when I talk to them? They don't, but I'm persistent. You see, I don't give up. That's what we all have in common here, Ms. Tilden. We don't give up, and we care about each other. We look after each other. Is that a new idea for you, Ms. Tilden? Helping someone else without being told to? 'Cause it's pretty fundamental here. No one is over and above anyone else here. Do you understand? Doctors are no better than anybody else. Your job is important, yes, but not more important than that of anyone else. Get it? We're about each other. We respect the role we each have here and the input we supply. Can you live with that?"

"I think so."

"Good, 'cause we need you. Ever been needed before? Ms. Tilden? I mean really needed?"

"No, I don't think that I ever have, frankly," Gail answered quietly.

"Ms. Tilden, why don't you follow me into my office and we'll talk a bit more." McClaren made no comment as the two of them walked through the darkened sanctuary and down the hall to his office. As they entered, McClaren indicated a chair for Gail. She sat down and watched McClaren go around his desk and sit down.

"So, Ms. Tilden let me welcome you again. Your resume looks great. How did you find us?"

"Oh, I had been doing some work for a person named Marcie Geck," Gail Tilden lied. "She seemed happy with my abilities and asked if I would like to spend some time in outcountry. Naturally, I was interested. I figured a change would do me good."

"That may be, or you might find outcountry unbearable Ms. Tilden." McClaren had noticed the young lady's neatly manicured hands. The simple beige suit matched her carefully almond streaked hair. "But we certainly need you. The government is using new encrypting methods, and we're having trouble keeping up. We really hope you can be of service there. We have good people here Ms. Tilden. Both the patients and the healthcare givers. We really have a good thing going. It's all confidential of course under cover of being a church," he paused, "which by the way, we really are. Have a congregation and everything. Maybe you would honor me by coming to one of the services sometime?" McClaren's bushy white eyebrows lifted with the questioning tone in his voice, his clear blue eyes gazing intently, so that Gail had to lower her own.

Ms. Tilden squirmed in her seat a bit. She had expected the Underground to be weird. But this man, McClaren, seemed normal except for this one thing, this religion thing. It simply wasn't done anymore. She didn't want to irritate him, but she didn't think she could pull off a pretend spirituality. She didn't know what spirituality looked like.

"We'll see. I'm not much for churches," she answered slowly, "and it's not because of the government," she hastily added. "It's just not for me, I guess. Hope you're not offended."

"Oh, not at all. I learned long ago to accept rejection. I've become quite good at it, naturally, living in the society we do. Most of the people downstairs in the hospital would agree with you. They just use me for the facility, and I allow them to do just that. Ever the optimist, I keep hoping someday just one will come around to my way of thinking. Just one would be fulfilling. Enough! Let's go meet the staff. We'll start with the office, then the medical staff. We all work together here and get on quite well, I'd say."

# CHAPTER 15

Marcie Geck had decorated her apartment in stark contrast to her no nonsense approach to life. She often splurged for extras when it came to her residence. She cared diligently for her plants. She had her little sketches and photos, that she created herself, framed and hung so that no wall was bare. Very different from most homes she went into. It looked homey she thought as she glanced around just before leaving to visit Matthew Salmund. He would be surprised, she knew, if he saw her place. Everyone thought she was so tough. Like that John Macklin character. She knew she scared him. She stopped as she went to pick up her shoulder bag. He was really kind of cute. Now why was she even thinking about him? He couldn't possibly be right for her. But still. He seemed to be an orphan. She knew what that meant. Wait. She couldn't weaken and let men enter into her thought process. Marcie worked hard at establishing and maintaining a tough image. She survived because of it. Loneliness provides motivation for so many things and protection from many people, she thought. Hadn't she created her own world? A safe haven from out there. A retreat. She found people interesting, but only allowed herself to observe—not to connect. And she believed in the work that she did. If she was to continue to provide an important service to society, she had to survive, and survival depended on skill, impartiality, and judgment.

Sleep just hadn't come for Marcie last night. She tried all of her regular tricks. Relaxation techniques, a trip to the kitchen, downloading a movie, nothing would do it. Odd for Marcie who slept anywhere, anytime, no problem. This meant something was troubling her, but what was it? Finally, giving up on sleep, Marcie had gone for an early morning run down the bike path that surrounded her living quarters, and halfway home, suddenly, a face had popped into her brain. An unfamiliar face but one that she knew she had met before. Just couldn't think at first. She stopped and sat down on one of the benches. Did some stretching exercises and got up to finish her run when she remembered. Matthew's office. Some starchy looking young woman in a surveillance photo Matthew showed her. Wanted an OK on her. What was her name? What had she wanted again? Oh yeah. The information was that she had found her way underground through Chuck Waller. Who did he know that Marcie didn't? Well, lots of suppliers for instance, she thought. But this gal was too upscale for the likes of him. If Marcie wanted to sleep tonight, she knew what she had to do. She had to find Waller and talk to him herself. Find out why he vouched for this person.

To that end, Marcie had put on her slumming clothes. Dirty jeans, oversized sweatshirt and a gun. She hardly ever carried, but, maybe it was her uneasiness, or maybe it was just the lack of sleep. She didn't know. But she breathed a sigh of relief as she placed it in her holster and headed out the door.

Food and slime attracted the Chuck Wallers of the world and that was exactly how Marcie found him. He was eating an overstuffed sandwich, drinking a beer, and sitting down at the filthy end of the harbor. "The dumping zone" as it was fondly referred to by the hobos of this area. Waller reminded her of a toad sitting on the edge of one of the pilings.

She had spotted him before he saw her, so engrossed in his sandwich was he.

"Hi Waller!"

"Why Marcie!" Waller immediately felt the hair on his neck rise. "What are you doing in these parts? Why didn't you contact me the usual way?"

"Oh, I wanted to surprise you," she said sweetly. "Besides, you apparently have another form of connecting that I don't know about. Maybe you could fill me in?"

The mental tapes of the last few days were rolling madly through Chuck's head. He tried to remember what he had done to produce the strident Marcie standing before him disturbing his lunch. He looked at her face and knew she was angry, but had no idea why. No idea at all. He slowly gulped the last of his sandwich and washed it down with the beer he had been holding in his left hand all the while. No idea why. He contemplated hitting Marcie over the head with the beer bottle, once he had finished the beer, of course, but then decided against it. Because of Marcie's connections, he made a lot of money.

"Well, I'm waiting."

"I really don't know what could be upsetting you, Marcie, my girl." It never hurt to try sweetness. "I've been sitting here most of the time catching up with my friends."

"Does the name, Tilden, mean anything to you?" she asked

"Tilden, Tilden. Nope," he replied happily. "You've got the wrong man." Marcie pulled out a picture and shoved it right into Waller's face. "Her!" And Marcie, seeing the look of recognition in Waller's eyes, gave him a shove. "Well, what do you know? You messed up. Again. She says you, of all people, vouched for her. Waller, you know you're not supposed to do that sort of thing. You know this, but look what you've done. Don't you like doing business with me and Salmund? Huh? What's the deal here? You should've come to us with this—not left us out. Now tell me, what did she say and what did you do?"

"It was nothing, just a sad story. She's lookin' for her hubby, that's all. Just that. Don't get all mad over nothing now. She looked dumb, you know, like she didn't know anything. She just wanted to find her husband, and, you know, I'm a nice guy, and I felt sorry for her so I just kind of suggested she head to outcountry."

"And just because we're such good friends and all, tell me how did you know about that?"

"Marcie, Marcie! Do you think I'm stupid? You're not my only dealer you know. I talk to other people—most of them are nicer to me than you are."

"Where?"

"Hmmm. I have friends all over the place—specially … "

"No! Stop!" Marcie yelled. "I don't want to hear about your connection with the Black Market; I just want to know where in outcountry did she go?" Marcie moved in closer to Waller. "Which place? Which place did she go to? I want to know now, Waller, 'cause I wonder if my people are safe. And then I want to know how much money she gave you. And was the money fresh or dirty?"

"Well," he admitted slowly, "it was pretty clean. I took it to my usual laundry, and he said no problem, came from an OK place," Waller looked around and let the words drop, "like a bank."

Marcie gasped. "Directly, Waller, directly? Think hard. Think. You know money straight from a bank can be government. You know that. Don't I pay you enough? Why did you have to take it, Waller? Now they know where you are."

"Naw, I'm OK. Nobody's been around, but thanks for the concern."

"Did you check her name out?"

"Well, I meant to, but I had other stuff to do. You know, you guys keep me pretty busy."

"Oh, OK, you listen real smart now. Don't call me for a while, not until I contact you again. You're tainted now. I'll use my other sources exclusively for a while. You wait for me to contact you. Stay away from me and Matthew."

"You protecting your boyfriend, now?" Waller couldn't resist. They had to be doing it. Marcie pretended not to hear or to care and hurried away, headed for Universal Health Club. This was bad. Matthew was not going to be at all happy about this. Who was this Tilden girl? Government. She could smell it.

She didn't wait for an announcement. Marcie barged into Salmund's office; Matthew looked up in surprise. Marcie walked directly up to his desk and stopped before him saying, "The system's tainted. What are we gonna do?" Matthew didn't like messes. She knew that about him. But he was methodical. She watched now as he carefully adjusted the papers he'd been working on. Once done, he looked up.

"Sit down, Marcie. And slow down. Would you like some coffee?" he asked in an attempt to calm her. She shook her head silently. "Now what do you know?"

"Not a whole lot." She filled him in on her visit to Waller.

"You know you have to stop using Waller?"

"I know."

"Maybe you should cool it for a while, too."

"Yeah, I know. I've gotta stay low. Actually, I was thinking that I might help best by going out to St. Luke's to warn them. I don't trust other forms of communication. Do you?"

"No, not really. But Marcie, this is dangerous. If it's government, you're in grave danger just being there. Remember, they have guns."

"Well, I have one, too."

"Aw, no, don't tell me that kind of stuff," Matthew groaned. "You know not to say something like that in my office." She held up her sweatshirt so he could see the pistol she had concealed in a holster. He grimaced.

"Go home. Right now. I'll call you. Let you know somehow what I want. And stop that defiant act. It's only going to get you in trouble, jail or worse. Then who would come here to torment me?"

"Matthew, is that a joke?" an incredulous Marcie reacted in spite of herself. Matthew smiled. Well, he had almost smiled.

# CHAPTER 16

"What a mess!" Marcie thought, as she rushed back to her apartment, found some ammo for her gun (in the back of her closet under her box of rarely used evening shoes) and dressed in her normal clothes. Pantsuit, comfortable shoes. Into her backpack she stuffed overnight toiletries and a change of clothes. As soon as she had arrived home, she had received an email from Matthew tersely worded. Within an hour she found herself with Matthew in a new car driving out of the city to outcountry. Matthew didn't talk, and she didn't want to irritate him, so she said nothing until they were out of the city.

"I'm sorry. This is my fault. I let you down. I know you don't like being away from the health center."

"Don't blame yourself," he said with no emotion.

"Well, I do."

"Well, don't. If it's anybody's fault, it's mine. I can't have more people dying on my watch."

"Oh yeah, Christiane." she said with a sigh. The muscles in his face tightened, but he said nothing.

"Come on, Matthew, you know I was there. Besides. everybody knows. You're quiet about it. But your buddy, Paul, he's a reporter, remember? You can't get to be that unless you're a blabbermouth. He doesn't tell everybody, but a lot of the right people know. It's OK, really, OK?"

"Just talk about something else."

"OK. Are we gonna die today? How about that for different? I mean aren't we just driving into a trap? Won't the government have people armed? People all around. Shouldn't we be afraid?"

"You don't have to come," Matthew said. And he suddenly pulled the car over on the now deserted road. "You don't have to come."

"Oh, come off it. You know I'm not getting out of this car. I just think we should have a plan, that's all."

"We're going to church. It's Sunday morning. Don't they have service on Sunday morning?"

"Oh! I hadn't thought of that. Yes, they do." Whenever Matthew talked through his clenched teeth, Marcie knew to back off. So Marcie decided to rest her eyes awhile.

Once safely in her room (which really wasn't too bad she had to admit), Gail opened her laptop and found a hookup in the wall. She had to report in to her supervisor. She noticed a funny feeling in her stomach. What was that? An unfamiliar feeling. A new feeling. "What is this?" she wondered aloud. Could she possibly feel guilty about all this? Ridiculous. They are the criminals. This McClaren guy showed a flagrant disregard for the law. What would our world be if there were no rules governing its resources? Didn't he know that medical resources would have run out long before now if it weren't for government restriction? "The same for all" provided the only fair method of disseminating medical care in the modern world. The first twenty years of the millennium had proved that. Resources had been depleted almost entirely when Congress finally acted to equalize healthcare. If not for such legislation, the situation would become untenable. She began unpacking and put an encrypted short message through to her boss.

For once, she felt her work really meant something to the future of the world. Yes, Reverend McClaren, every person could contribute something vital to the world. And shutting you down will be my special role in society. Soon she would meet the rest of McClaren's band of merry thieves. That was all that they were. Stealing from the rest of society. What right did they have? They really belong in jail, she thought resolutely. A voice inside her quietly said, "Even John?"

She would keep her opinions to herself and just observe. Those were her orders. And she planned to follow them. At least for now. This job could finally give her career the push it needed.

The police car silently slithered up on the back bumper of Marcie and Matthew's car. They had been talking about nothing in particular, dazed by the glare of the sun and the long, boring drive. Suddenly, the siren on the car tailing them blared, and the two of them jumped.

"Should we try to lose them?" Marcie asked.

"Out here? Do we have a chance in this little thing? That police car has a lot more engine than this."

"Yeah, how we gonna play this?"

"Don't know."

"Let me take the rap for it. You just be dumb about everything. You're just out for a ride. I'll take the fall. The organization needs you more than me. And Matthew, you know that is true. I can be easily replaced. But not you."

The siren was insistent. Now the car tried to physically force them off the road.

"OK! OK! We're slowing down!" Marcie shouted. Their car puttered to a stop. Marcie took a deep breath and got out of the car to face the cops. How had this happened? Waller immediately came to mind. She never should have gotten mixed up with him. She knew that. Learning it the hard way.

She turned to face the cop and saw a familiar face! "I know you!" she shouted. Amazed, she asked, "What are you doing here?"

"Now the questions," Rufuos said slowly, leaning against his car, "they're my job. So just calm yourself down."

"You better show just cause for this stop. I know I have rights. You better not have just been bored today, Officer King."

"So, you know my name. That's refreshing. At least you're not pretending you don't know who I am. Just like I am not gonna pretend I don't already know you. I have a clear purpose for stopping you and your friend in there."

"He knows nothing about anything."

"Yeah, yeah, I know. It's nothing. He knows nothing. You just out for a Sunday drive. Well this Sunday is different 'cause I've got my nine year-old son in the car, and he needs what you can give him. So I guess you have a choice today, Ms. Geck, and that is to help me out or I am gonna bring you and your friends in for questioning or something. I'm real motivated today, Ms. Geck. And I have a real active imagination, so I'm sure I can come up with something." Rufuos felt the anger rise up from his gut like a snake looking for a way out of a cage.

Marcie looked beyond Rufuos to his car. "I don't see anyone."

"That's 'cause he's lying down. He's sick. Bad sick. Wellness Center can't help him. Say they phased out the drug that could have helped him a long time ago. Say it was getting too expensive. Too expensive! I figure I've given you some breaks. You know I have, so now I need a break from you, Ms. Geck. I need a way into the Underground. No way am I taking him to a Black Market doctor. And I'm gettin' desperate about it," he hissed. He paused, tried to pull himself together, "So what do you say? You gonna help or what?"

"I need to see the boy." Marcie said. She groaned inwardly, it had to be a kid. So they went over to take a look. Marcie glanced back at Matthew in the car watching her follow Officer King over to his police car. Officer King opened the back car door and Marcie ducked down to take a good look at the officer's son. The boy looked listlessly up at her. Marcie said nothing. She stood up and looked at Officer King.

"How do you know the medicine is manufactured anywhere?"

"I don't, but I figure I gotta do something to help him. He's my kid! You can understand, can't you?"

Marcie took a deep breath. "Let me go talk to Matthew."

Rufuos waited while Marcie returned to her car. She sat with Matthew for quite a while. Then the two of them came out. Matthew went to look at the child. Matthew was friendly with the kid. Then returned to Marcie and Rufuos.

"Here's the thing." Matthew began, "The place we're going to. We think the government is getting ready to seize that site. So we're really not sure if that's such a good idea for you. He looks pretty tired, but do you think he can make it to the next clinic?"

"Let's face it. Any place illegal is risky. I could get him all the way to the next hospital and find that one is crawling with government agents, too. Come on, I'm willing to give it a try. And I know he is."

"OK, how about this. You hang back. Let Marcie and me go in first. We'll check the place out and then get word to you. We know who we're looking for. And we're hoping the government has not sent more than the one agent at this point. Then maybe we can get your boy in and out fast, get him the meds he needs, and send him on home with you."

Rufuos' face showed sheer relief at knowing he had not failed, not yet anyway, in his quest for his son. He jumped back into his car turning once to check his son and then, looking ahead, waited to follow Marcie and Matthew's car.

Marcie and Matthew got back into their car.

"We have to just trust him," Matt said reasonably.

"I have a hard time with that."

"Me too," Matt turned to face Marcie, "but we have no choice and sometimes you just have to trust. It's the way, the only way we can keep our organization going. We have been lucky so far. But once in a while someone slips in. Besides, I can't refuse help to that boy."

"Matthew, you are just full of surprises. OK, I'm in." Marcie then chuckled quietly and said, "A police officer and one who has followed me, to boot. Well, maybe they're not all bad, and I'm sure they know that the commissioner and mayor and everybody above them get top tier care while the rest of us get the crumbs of what is left of the medical resources."

"Yeah, I know. If we can keep this quiet, maybe Rufuos King can be of future help to us."

"Oh right, what can he do for us?" Was Matt getting too soft?

"Protection, maybe, at times, I think, yes, he could be of use," Matthew said more to himself than to Marcie.

After getting settled in, Gail decided to be brave and venture out of her room. She wandered down to the main entrance where she had come in and found that church was over. Reverend McClaren, upon seeing her, smiled and said, "I hope you will be comfortable in your room."

"Oh, yes, it's fine. Much better than I expected. I mean it's fine," she stammered. "How was your, uh, talk?"

"Sermon, you mean."

"Yes, sermon."

"Actually, it went quite well. The five people sitting out there seemed to like it. I guess humility is something the Lord wants me to learn." McClaren smiled.

"I'm sure it was fine. Would you like to wait awhile or do you want to show me around now?"

"Now is good. Let me just drop some books off in the church office, and I'll be right with you." He returned shortly and said, "OK, here we go." You'll see that we don't have the best to offer in terms of a facility, but we really work hard to do a good job with our patients." He led Ms. Tilden through the dimly lit but immaculately clean sanctuary to a door located at the side and front of the church. He opened it to reveal a staircase down. Gail heard the noise of the hospital first. A gentle hum of equipment underscored the voices Gail heard even before they finished descending the stairs into the hospital.

McClaren talked as he walked pointing out various equipment and occasionally introducing Ms. Tilden to a medical caregiver.

"Why don't these patients just go to a regular Wellness Center?" Ms. Tilden asked.

"Well, of course, most of them have tried that already. Occasionally, we get someone who refuses to go to a government based hospital. But most people don't like to buck the system and actually do head for a government hospital first. Which is just as well 'cause we can't take care of everybody. We'd like to, of course, but it would be just impossible. So we provide care for those who have already met their quota and are going to be turned away by the government. Or we get people whose problem is just overlooked by the government techs. Then there are a few who come to us because of what I call libertarian leanings. They just want to feel in control of their destiny. I know it sounds provincial, but I respect those people." A buzzer sounded.

"That's the front door. Must be someone from the outside world. Gotta go. Here, Marilyn, could you take Ms. Tilden under your wing for a bit?"

Marilyn had just walked in the back door from the dormitory. She stopped and looked at Ms. Tilden, "Of course, I'll be happy to show you around."

"He rushed off a bit panicked," Ms. Tilden observed.

"He can't help feeling panicked whenever the outdoor buzzer rings unexpectedly," Marilyn smiled as she watched McClaren take the steps up to the sanctuary two at a time.

And this was definitely unexpected. McClaren had been aware of no special visits.

Marcie's gaze traveled up past the front door of the church all the way up to the steeple and back down again. She looked back at the car and then at Matthew standing by her side. Rufuos waited down the road in the direction from which they had come. Marcie could barely see him standing by his car.

"McClaren!" Marcie said a bit forcefully as the door opened.

"That's me."

"Remember me? Marcie Geck? And this is Matthew Salmund. He works with me in the city. You probably are a little surprised to see us."

"I certainly am, but everyone is welcome at St. Luke's," Reverend McClaren said unconvincingly.

"I have no doubt of that. We're here for just that reason. See, we're worried that you at present have a government agent undercover in your building. We'd hate to see your work jeopardized by such a person. We came by this information in an odd sort of way," Marcie thought of Waller. "We're not absolutely sure, so we thought we should come on down and see if we could work this out," Marcie continued.

"You do remember me, don't you? I brought you Chambers and Macklin? I procure drugs for you, and Matthew, he does just about everything to keep you outcountry clinics going. Oh and the password for today is resilience."

"I remember you. I just wasn't expecting anyone today," Reverend McClaren replied. "I think you had better come in. We'll talk in my office. Actually someone new did arrive today. Don't know if she's one of them or not. She came here to help with encryption. One of the doctors is down there showing her around right now." He closed the door behind them and paused. "I have never had a breach since St. Luke's started. Don't really know what to do even if this Ms. Tilden is a problem. What makes you suspect her?"

"Well, she used bank money to pay off an informant. None of us uses banks for anything. And it's an informant I don't trust."

"If she is, then what are we going to do?" McClaren asked anxiously as he guided the two into his office.

"Good question." Marcie said as she sat down. "We'll have to apprehend her. Don't know what we are gong to do about her. But we need to check her out."

"And how are we going to do that?"

Marcie paused and then turned to Matthew. "We can take her fingerprints to that computer nerd you use so much, Paul, and hack into the government fingerprint base." She thought a moment. "Yeah, that's what we'll do. He'll help us?" She looked questioningly at Matt.

"Sounds like a good idea to me. We need to have Paul's help with this."

"What if she is government?" McClaren asked looking from Marcie to Matt.

Matt looked directly into McClaren's eyes as he spoke, "In this business we figure things out as we go along, but we'll definitely have to do something to protect you, the staff, and your patients. These are hard decisions, but I don't think you're ready for your patients to become sacrificial lambs."

McClaren breathed deeply and said resignedly, "Definitely not. Of course, you're right. Let's see. She's the only new person in quite some time, so I guess if she turns out clean, we'll be out of the woods on this one, don't you think?"

"I agree," Matt answered. "Um, there is one other thing," he went on glancing at Marcie.

"What else?" McClaren asked exasperated.

"Actually this might be a little easier for you to handle since it is the reason you are here."

"And what is that?"

"Why to help people get well. That's right, isn't it?" Matt asked innocently.

McClaren answered, "Of course."

"OK then. It seems we have another patient for you. He's young, nine years old."

"Well, naturally, bring him to us," McClaren interrupted enthusiastically.

"Ah, there is one thing you should know," Marcie interceded. Before McClaren said anything, she went on, "Aaron, that's the patient's name. Aaron is very ill and wants your help and so does his dad. Only thing you should know is his father is a police officer with the government." She stopped and allowed McClaren time to take in this new information.

"Well, what sort of attitude does this police officer have toward us here at St. Luke's? Is this just a come on? I know I'm a minister, and people think they can just do anything around me, but even I have my limits."

"I actually think you will be OK with Rufuos King. I think he is quite desperate really. He told me he hasn't told his partner or anyone else at the police station."

"If you think it's OK." McClaren gazed down the road. "We'll take care of him."

Marcie smiled and jumped up, "I'll just go give them the good news," she said. Matthew's gaze followed her out the door in wonder.

# CHAPTER 17

Many who ventured to outcountry would drive right past St. Luke's without even noticing it. It stood, a fruit tree gone barren, only as testimony to history now forgotten. Who even thought about religion anymore? Certainly no one missed it. Probably St. Luke's structure dated to the early nineteenth century. Its white frame exterior now graying and faded due to nature and time simply reminded those who happened by to notice that a few old things remained. One expected such sights in outcountry. They meant nothing.

Perhaps churches then served best as cover for the Underground medical facilities they now housed. Few government officials had made the connection. Science just didn't accept mythology (now considered synonymous with the twentieth century popular religions).

While the outside of St. Luke's remained somewhat shody, the inside provided stark contrast. The pews were dusted regularly (and restained as required) sustained by the efforts of the church pastor, Reverend McClaren, who adhered to a regular schedule of painting (the walls), and scrubbing the floor, an ancient linoleum of dull brown. These duties provided therapy, while serving as a reminder of his own humble station in the world.

McClaren definitely had a constant struggle with pride. His mind turned over the problem of pride, the teachings of the Bible. The conflict between pride and humility had never been fully resolved in his own mind. Servitude seemed to matter; thus, the paintbrush and mop.

After the dimness of the sanctuary, Ms. Tilden squinted at the brightness of the hospital. The room, historically, had been a large meeting hall. It now was an amazingly well equipped hospital. Gail stood for a very long time, stunned by the magnitude of what had been done here. At the end of the corridor stood a very traditional looking nurses station. Marilyn motioned her to follow. As they walked down the hall, Gail peeked into the rooms on either side and saw patients in hospital beds surrounded by modern equipment. Marilyn stopped at one door.

"Come on in. Meet one of my favorites."

Gail timidly entered.

"Hi, Ben. Meet Gail." A young man taking the patient's blood pressure looked up and nodded.

"So you're here to torture me again!" This, from the patient, an elderly man with a full beard and long white hair.

Marilyn laughed. "No, not this time, Mr. Miller. Just thought I'd bring a pretty lady here, so you could maybe remember what class looks like."

"I've got you, ain't I?"

"You're such a man—how could I possibly satisfy you totally?"

He glanced at Gail and looked over at Marilyn.

"No, seriously. The pain is bad, Doc. Real bad. These meds this kid, Ben, is giving me, they work for a while, but when they wear off, it's holy hell for me."

Ben handed Marilyn the chart. "I've been giving him what you ordered."

"I know. I think we need to increase it a bit." She handed the chart back to Ben and went over and took Mr. Miller's hand. "I'm ordering you more pain medicine. Just holler for Ben if it isn't enough, and he'll come get me. Right, Ben?" She looked over at him.

"You got it," he answered.

Marilyn smiled at Mr. Miller. "And stop staring at Ms. Tilden. You're getting yourself all worked up. What about Mrs. Miller?"

"Aw, she don't care, long as I tell her she can be the boss, she don't care."

"Right. Sure. Your wife is a stunner, and you know it. I'm off now, but you behave for Ben."

"Sure, sure, he's young. I'll get him trained for you, Doc."

"Yeah, Mr. Miller, but can you find a hottie for him?"

Mr. Miller turned his attention to Ben. "Aw, forget it, kid. I ain't no miracle worker. Now shoot me some of that good stuff Dr. Marilyn told me I could have."

Marilyn and Gail had moved down the hall to the nurse's station where Marilyn picked up some more patient charts.

"Aren't you worried about overdosing him? And doesn't some-one have to review your orders?" Gail asked.

Marilyn looked up from the chart she was reading,
"Review?"

"Right. In the government hospitals they have a review, so mis-takes are not made."

"Really? I guess we don't need that here. There are so many care-givers seeing the patients that we catch each other's mistakes, or we make suggestions regarding the patient's care. We don't need a formal review." She closed the chart and turned to face Gail. "Review. Hmmm. Isn't that code for 'disallow' out in that world?"

Gail just stared. "No, I don't think so," her voice faded away.

"Really? Ms. Tilden, Mr. Miller is dying. He knows it. His wife knows it. We all know it. But we are not going to allow him to suffer if we can help it. What good are all these advances if we can't use them to alleviate pain and suffering? If we had a review, the kind you're talking about, Mr. Miller would not be getting the medicine he is getting. In fact, he wouldn't be allowed to get anything. I'm sure, according to government standards, he used up his allotment a long time ago. Some diseases just can't be cured. At least, not yet. Mr. Mil-ler has pancreatic cancer. He has pain. Pain I really can't imagine, but I have to believe him when he tells me, and I don't need a review board to tell me. Does he look like a complainer to you?"

Tilden shook her head.

"No. He's not. I am here to help him on his way to the end. If I can't cure him, I can at least allow him the dignity of being pain free so that he can spend quality moments with his wife."

Tilden decided to change the subject, "How did you get all these computers. They look like government issue. How can this be?"

"We do have all the latest in computer technology, which pro-vides the medical staff with any information one would find in a government facility." Marilyn ran her hand over the nearest machine, which happened to be monitoring a patient's heart. Are you im-pressed?"

"Well, I suppose. I don't see how you could have accumulated so much here." Gail moved from one computer to the next. There were five in all. "Also, your people working the computers actually know what they are doing. Where did they train? The government does not share its information technology with private sources."

"That's precisely why we need you, Ms Tilden." Our people had to figure things out for themselves. With your help our computers will be a lot more useful."

"Right, of course," Gail answered.

"We could have gone to the Black Market and paid a hefty fee to get the information you are going to help us with," Marilyn said.

There it was again. The Black Market. Gail's face must have shown confusion since Marilyn continued, "The Black Market is a totally separate organization. One we frown on, by the way."

"I don't have any idea what you are talking about. I thought this was the Black Market."

"No," Marilyn replied, "We are the Underground. Huge difference. We provide help to any and all. We don't blackmail people, and we don't threaten them. We ask only for donations. Believe it or not, we always have enough. We believe all are entitled to medical care. Let me re-say that, the best medical care. Here's the deal. In the city, people have government-supplied healthcare. Healthcare which is limited because of funds or supply of medicines or supply of doctors—all resources that are hard to come by these days; therefore, government patients receive only what we here at St. Luke's would consider minimal care. Just like at other Underground facilities, we try to overcome such limits. We think creatively about health problems. We don't turn people away simply because they have had the bad luck of being born with many health problems. So we are constrained by some of the same limitations the government agencies have, but we try to find ways to circumvent such limits. The government, in its effort to be totally fair, ends up being totally unfair. Further, it fosters the growth of the Black Market. The Black Market works only for profit. Prices for all care in the Black Market are exorbitant. A patient can obtain any type of healthcare if he can pay the price. Black Market doctors treat all, but, unfortunately, do not maintain any set of standards. No one cares about failed treatments, much like the government health program. Good healthcare requires time, a resource I didn't mention before, but a resource all the same. Here we have reverted to medicine as it was practiced in the middle of the twentieth century, with one big difference. We use all modern technology and treatments available." Marilyn watched Gail carefully. "Have I thrown too much at you today?"

"No, not at all."

"Hmm. You haven't really convinced me. Let's just go finish my rounds. Then I'll give you time to wander around by yourself." They continued room by room. Gail stood back and just watched. She couldn't believe she had actually pulled off this ruse. She kept a calm look on her face, but inside she bursted to tell someone. Couldn't wait to get back to her room to report in. She started daydreaming about how to spend the nice bonus she would get for this.

"I think you have seen it all at this point." Marilyn came to a stop out in the hall after visiting the last patient, "What do you think?"

"I think what you have done here is remarkable," Gail lied.

"I appreciate that. I think it's important for you to understand how important our work is here and how your computer knowledge will enable better care for the people here."

"I'm glad to be a part of this." Gail couldn't wait to relay all this good stuff to her superior. She had heard enough sob stories to last her a lifetime. The patients they had visited each told his or her story of frustration with the government source of medical care. Marilyn thanked each one before moving on. Some were bitter. Others resigned to their situation. Gail had said nothing.

"Naturally, I can see why you're excited about what you do, Marilyn. Isn't it scary for you, though?"

"No, not really." Marilyn ran her hand through her wavy honey brown hair. Her brown eyes surveyed the hospital hall then came to rest on Gail. "I guess if I really stop and think too much about what I am doing here, I would get scared. But out there was scary too. Here, I'm with people I trust. They really care about me. We look out for each other. The patients feel the same way, I believe. You'll get used to it here."

"I'm sure I will," Gail replied. She believed she had convinced Marilyn of her sincerity.

"You know, having you here, Gail, will help enormously. I'm sure we'll all be somewhat safer with you working on the computer system. Let's see. Is there anything else I should show you? A lot of our staff has gone on what we like to call a shopping trip. We had gotten dangerously low on some basic meds such as antibiotics and steroids. You'll get to meet them all tomorrow."

"I don't have any questions right now. If you're through with me for now, I could use a bit of a rest before dinner. I need some time to absorb all this." Shopping trip. Must be their euphemism for stealing.

"Right," Marilyn smiled. "Just head straight down that hall and you'll see the door to the outside and the dorm just beyond. Dinner's at seven. See you there."

"Yeah, thanks, and thanks for the tour."

"No problem. We're glad to have you here." Marilyn watched as Ms. Tilden took one last look around and then left.

Gail Tilden headed across the gravel parking lot (with only one ancient car in it) to the building referred to as the dorm. She didn't know if they expected her to start work today or not. But she needed to be alone. And she needed to make contact with her supervisor. What would she do next? And, she hadn't seen John anywhere. Did that change things for her? Would she stay anyway? Or head off to look for him. Did she miss him at all, she wondered. The sun felt warm after the artificial light in the hospital basements where she had spent most of her day. As she stumbled across to the dorm building, she heard a little beep and saw an approaching car. She looked up tentatively trying to spy the driver behind the dusty windshield, but she really could see nothing. She gave a shy wave and headed to her room.

"Who's that?!" John gasped from the passenger seat of the car. He felt his stomach lurch as his brain processed what he had just seen.

"Don't know. McClaren did say he was expecting someone today," Chambers responded as he parked the car.

"Oh no! It can't be. I'm so sunk. So completely sunk! You are all gonna hate me." John turned in his seat to watch the woman enter the dorm. "It just can't be. I cannot believe this is happening."

"What? What is it? What are you babbling about?"

"It's her! I know it can't be, but it looks just like her. Who were they expecting today? Do you know? I've got to see McClaren right now." He tugged at the door handle, threw the supplies that were sitting on his lap onto the car seat, and ran to the main building heading first to the sanctuary.

"McClaren! McClaren! I need to speak to you right now! McClaren, where are you?" No sign of him, no lights on. Maybe his office. John started down the hall away from the sanctuary when he heard McClaren. He stopped, turned around, and walked back into the sanctuary. McClaren sat in the dark in the second pew.

"Here I am. Calm down now, John. What can I do for you? Just calm down."

John couldn't speak. He stopped and leaned over hands on knees in an attempt to clear his head. He had difficulty getting the words out.

"What do you want to say?" Reverend McClaren spoke softly. And then gently, "What can I do for you? No, wait, first come sit down here."

John felt the nausea recede. He stood up slowly. His face still felt clammy, but he successfully made it over to where McClaren sat.

McClaren patted him on the shoulder as he sat down next to him. "I just sit here sometimes in the dark. Seems I can see more clearly that way." McClaren said nothing for a while. "Now what is this fuss about?"

"Your guest," John gasped. "Who is she? Why is she here?"

"We needed some help with the computers. Actually, I don't know how long she will work here. It really won't affect you. At least not directly."

"What's all this about?" Chambers asked panting from the exertion of running after John.

John knew he had to keep himself together. His hands involuntarily fished around in his pocket. Oh right, no pills. He somehow found the resolve to speak, "What is the woman's name?" John asked McClaren.

"Gail Tilden."

"Oh great." Chambers sat down in the pew behind them. "Just great."

"I know, I know. It's not good. What are we going to do?" John looked at McClaren.

"Hmm. She did only just arrive. Why don't we all stay calm," McClaren said.

Maybe he could be calm and maybe Chambers could, but not John. "It's just this. She is my wife!" And here he paused, drew a deep breath and went on bravely, "My wife works. You know this already. She works for the government, you know, The U.S. Healthcare Delivery System. She shuts places like this down. Or at least she would if she could," he said. "Right now, I don't know exactly what she is doing 'cause I left home, remember?"

"Oh yeah, we remember," Chambers responded sarcastically. "I can't believe you could be this stupid. You led her right to us. She's the same woman who came to my house to investigate me."

"Now, Dr. Chambers," McClaren interjected. "Let's see if we can reason this out first before pointing a finger of blame." He gave Chambers a stern look. "I think the two of you should come to my office. I have some guests waiting there."

As Chambers and John entered ahead of McClaren, they saw Marcie and Matthew talking quietly looking at a laptop computer screen.

Marcie turned abruptly when she heard them enter and addressed John. "You! What's going on? Have you been making trouble here?"

John tried to breathe normally and replied, "No, this was the best move I ever made. I like it here. Plus, I am learning stuff I never knew anything about. I feel like I'm helping, most of the time, just not right now."

"Now, now, don't be too hard on yourself," McClaren said. "Please just sit down and tell all of us what's going on."

"The new computer person is my wife. My wife!"

"We know." This from Marcie and Salmund simultaneously.

"You already know?" John looked from one to the other. "When were you going to tell me? She is gonna kill me."

"It's not you we're worried about." Marcie tried to maintain her composure. "We need you to tell us everything. Everything about her."

"Well, OK. I never paid too much attention to her job. You know she works for the government in one of the Healthcare System Divisions?" John paused as realization struck and then, "Oh yeah! Oh, I mean no! She isn't really here for me."

McClaren held a chair for John to sit. Then, "We think she is here to investigate us. And we want to know all you can tell us. Then we're gonna figure out what to do."

"I think I'm gonna be sick." John dropped his head down between his legs. What a disaster, he thought, and then said aloud to no one in particular, "This could have been so great for me. Now SHE is here to ruin it all."

Marcie stood up and walked over to John, "You can see, John, we're in a bit of a pickle. Now we don't want her to leave—not just yet anyway. We could find out some stuff, you know. And that's where you come in."

"Yeah, John, here's your chance to pay them back, to get back at The System that has used you. Think about it." Dr. Chambers joined in.

"I don't know. I'm not good at stuff like this—hard nose kind of stuff where I could get in deep trouble. And Gail. She can be very stubborn. She thinks her job is so-o-o important. But she never really told me what she does there."

"Is she good with computers?" This from McClaren.

"Oh yeah, she took care of all of ours at home. Always made fun of me and how I didn't know much about the insides."

"How high-level is she?"

"That's what's strange about all this. I thought she was low level. You know, never this kind of underground work. Just a pencil pusher, I think they call 'em. And audits. She did audits."

"Like for physicians operating outside The System?" Chambers spoke up.

"Yeah, just like that. She never found anyone though. She wanted to, that's for sure. Always talked about how she wanted that first break."

"Well, I guess that's what we are, Ms. Tilden's first break." McClaren breathed deeply and looked up momentarily.

"So, she *is* my wife. Maybe she is here to find me?" Could it be that she really did care about him and their marriage?

"Oh, you're going to get a chance to ask her," McClaren said. "We're just gonna do a little orchestrating."

"Could we all be connected with her?" Chambers asked looking at Marcie and Matthew. "I'm here because of someone like her."

"What was the agent's name who came to your house?" McClaren asked.

"Don't know, don't remember. But I would know her if I saw her. She stayed long enough."

"OK, here's what we'll do. We're going to make sure she sits with you all at dinner. We'll see how she decides to act. Is she gonna fess up to being John's wife? Perhaps she knows no one? Course John, you're going to skip dinner tonight. We're keeping you under wraps until we can tell what she is up to. She will have to admit it if she knows Chambers. She'll have to come up with some sort of a story. We'll let her squirm a bit. Maybe we can figure out what she is up to—is she simply looking for John or does she have other plans? But she still won't know that you are here. We want to watch her and get information first before we show our cards. Hopefully, no one else is coming. They have to gather written evidence first. That's what she'll be doing first. So we have some time before the Feds turn up with their tanks and stuff."

Startled, Macklin looked up. Tanks! "What's the worst case scenario?"

McClaren rested his hand on John's shoulder, "We won't discuss that right now. We'll just say that Plan B will be to evacuate to another station. I'm going to have to contact several other sites to see if we can get the vehicles here. That's the problem always, transportation. As many patients as we can, we send home—that's what we'll do. The serious ones require serious solutions. We'll figure it out. Have faith."

"Yeah," John said, "Faith. Keep hearing that word lately. Guess I'll figure out eventually what it means."

McClaren glanced at John and then the others. "I'm going to talk to the people in the dining room about seating. For now, everybody just continue normally. I'm going to check online and see if there is anything of note about Ms. Tilden. Maybe see what she's about."

Ms. Tilden had hurried into her room and, though she should have been tired, her excitement had taken over. She started her wireless communiqué with a rundown on what she had seen today. He would be happy, she thought. 'Course she didn't tell him everything. Everything would be too much. She might be able to sell the information later to a news agency or something. She was a bit worried about her own safety, too. What if the Feds descend on this place with gas and tanks? Would they give her advance warning, so she could get out? It scared her to be in a situation, new and dangerous. But at the same time, it was kind of fun. Life, up to now, had been a bore, and medical espionage, as long as she didn't get hurt, could turn out to be a fun diversion. She hoped so anyway. The people here were like at home, boring. But she would shake the place up a bit, she thought. This could turn out to be, at the very least, interesting.

Even not finding John didn't seem like a big thing anymore. Time to move on. Forget him, just get divorced and look for someone new. Maybe someone in the Central Government, someone with money and prestige. That would be really nice.

# CHAPTER 18

Meanwhile McClaren contacted his colleagues at other Underground hospital sites. No one had heard of Ms. Tilden. He had weighed the risk of communicating online and had decided if there was a breach, it had happened already. He needed to set up a plan if this deceitful woman, Tilden, was to be confronted. He needed to make plans for his people, the sick and the healthy. They were his responsibility. They had trusted him. And McClaren took such trust very seriously.

But for now he would have dinner. Usually on time, he sauntered in late.

"Hello, everyone!" He greeted them with smiles. "Ms. Tilden, so glad to have you here." He pulled his chair back, sat down and placed his napkin in his lap. "You all by now have met Ms. Tilden, right?" He smiled over at her seated to his right. She looked decidedly uncomfortable. "Hmmm, won't someone let me in on the topic of conversation. You all are uncharacteristically quiet."

Chambers spoke up never taking his eyes off of Gail. "We were just talking about why someone who investigates doctors who are outside the System would want to suddenly help a whole gosh darn hospital."

"Dr. Chambers, no need to raise your voice." Reverend McClaren turned to Ms. Tilden, "Why are you here?"

"I'm looking for my husband."

"Really?" Marilyn said. "That's all there is to it? You walked around here like you were so interested. Wasted my time. Time I could have spent with patients. You wanted to know everything." She looked over at McClaren, "What are we going to do with her?"

Gail's eyes darted around involuntarily checking out the nearest exit.

McClaren said. "You are not going anywhere just yet, Ms. Tilden. We will decide when you may leave."

The color left Gail's face as she realized she no longer had control. She placed her fork on her plate. "What are you going to do to me?"

McClaren answered, "We haven't figured that out yet. Don't worry, we don't treat people who oppose us in the same manner your government does. There will be no mind numbing medicines and no jail, although we will keep you here. You will be under, I guess what you would call, house arrest while we sort this out. Your presence makes our lives very difficult and even will affect the care of our patients. He looked at the others. I'm leaning toward having her help us. You know, assist in whatever way she is able."

"I won't do it."

"Of course, you can choose to resist, Ms. Tilden, but I think someone like you might want to get a feel for everything we do here, so that when you return to your world of corruption, you will have lots to say and sell. That is what this is about, isn't it? You might even change your mind about a few things."

"You will not be able to change me. My mind is fine without your hocus pocus or whatever it is you do."

"Oh, Ms. Tilden, you think you hurt me by saying such things? Forget it. I've heard it all before, even from some of my good friends sitting here. You will not change me. Our lives, however, are now linked, whether that is what you intended or not."

"This is ridiculous!" Gail stood up abruptly, causing her chair to fall backward to the floor. "You are all criminal hypocrites! You can twist it all you want, but this hospital is illegal, and you are all breaking the law!" No one said a word. In fact, they followed Reverend McClaren's lead and calmly continued their dinner.

Frustrated, Gail turned and left. Calmly, to let them know they had not gotten to her. But they had. As she walked back to her room, disturbing thoughts came to mind. Could she be subverted to their way of thinking? Of course not! She pouted a bit and then smiled. She was stronger than everyone thought. She had proved that already!

Once finally in her room, Gail decided she needed to sleep. Her eyes had been drooping so she finally succumbed and flopped across the bed falling into a delightful sleep where fantasies of her career exploits entertained. She dreamed of the new titles she would have once she finished her business at St. Luke's. Perhaps a judgeship would follow. She would handle the gavel of justice with fairness and wisdom. Her dream ceased with the heavy knocking on her door. It took her a minute to realize where she was.

All thoughts of joy disappeared as she reached for her shoes and announced, "Please come in."

The door opened slowly and, to her amazement, her husband, John, stood before her.

"You!" Somehow he seemed older and even handsomer. Had they only been apart a few days?

"So it is you," he said quietly.

"What do you mean? Of course, it's me. I had to find you, didn't I?"

"Actually, I'm kind of surprised you even came looking for me."

"Well, I had to, didn't I? What would people think?"

"Oh right. Here we go. What would they think, Gail? Let me see, 'John being John again. Your joke of a husband just being his usual self. Irresponsible, deficient John. Don't want him out there running loose. Don't know what might happen to poor John.'"

Gail's face reddened. Had she really thought he was that stupid?

"So, I have that much right, don't I?"

Gail fidgeted. "Stop staring. You're making me uncomfortable. And why shouldn't I be angry? You left me! Left me! Not a word." Had he been working out? He stood up straight with shoulders squared. His eyes, once constantly averted, made direct contact with hers. After a pause, Gail stepped forward to give him a rather chaste hug. He didn't hug back. For his part, he wondered if he had ever cared about her.

"Aren't you just a little bit happy to see me?" No answer. "Well, if you have to think about it that hard, I guess that's my answer." She pretended to be sad.

"Come on. Admit it. You were relieved when you saw I was gone. You're just using me as an excuse to get in with these people. You can just forget that. They are onto you!"

"I already know that. Do you think I'm stupid? They're actually holding me here. Listen, I could get you out of here." She reached over and ran her hand gently down his arm. "I could still do it, John. Especially if you were to give me some inside information. That would really help you, John."

"Help me? Hell, it would help you and only you, and maybe a few people up the ladder in the government. I wonder if it would help you. You think your supervisor cares about you? Think again, little girl. That's what you are and always will be, a little girl. And you are going to be in over your head on this one. Way over." He watched her cower.

"Maybe you're right about that. Maybe they don't care about me, but I care about my job, and I thought you cared about yours. I don't see how you could be a part of this, John. And I don't know how you could have just run off and left me."

John sighed and went over to sit next to her on the bed.

"I didn't plan it. It just happened. I got into a little trouble at the Wellness Center, and I didn't want you to be pulled down with me. So I escaped the city and came out here. They need me here. You never needed me except to fill the seat next to you at those boring office dinners of yours. I'm nothing to you." John stopped and looked at her directly. "Come on, admit it. We never had a real marriage, just more like an agreement. Like business partners."

"I suppose you're right. Just business partners. I will miss you at those dinners though." She looked away and seemed to be talking more to herself than to John. "You must have been so bored. All that educated talk."

"Oh right!" John angrily interrupted her musings. "There you go with your attitude. That attitude that says you're better than me," John paused. "Wait a minute. You're better than everyone," he hissed and then yelled, "especially me. Isn't that right?" John moved closer. "Isn't that what you really think?"

John halted. Had he actually stood up to Gail? She had a perplexed look on her face. They were both stunned by this new John. Where had he come from? And where was the guy who couldn't handle the slightest upsets in life? Sure, he was shaking all over but still, he had stood up to her.

"Well, I guess you've changed," Gail said. "Didn't know you had any guts at all, John. Don't know how I feel about you now. Actually, I'm thinking I may like this new John better." She crossed over to him and put her arms around him. He carefully pulled them away and walked over to the door. He looked back at her.

"I'm not a machine that you can turn on and off." He paused. "Forget us for a moment. Tell me. What are you doing here? Why did you come here?"

"Why, to find you, of course. I was actually missing you." Gail looked at him with her most sincere face.

"How did I ever fall for you?" John asked in wonder.

"Oh, thanks a lot." She sat down on the bed arms folded.

"What did you think when you found me? That I would just fol-low you home? Even if I wanted to for your sake, I don't have a job anymore. Remember? I'm wanted by the U.S. Government. Probably by your agency. Is that why you followed me? To make the great coup you've always hoped for. To finally show your parents you're not just a pencil pusher?"

"Are you on some new medicine that I don't know about," Gail sputtered in surprise.

He laughed at her confusion.

"Don't know where all this bravado is coming from." She pouted. "But, no, I'm here because my supervisor sent me," she lied. "Finding you makes for an added bonus. But I didn't really know where you had gone."

"Listen Gail, you can't turn this place in." John decided to change his tactic. "Please. Let me show you around."

"I've had the tour, thank you. You're quite an altruistic bunch. I'll give you that. But that doesn't mean I can ignore what is happening here. It's totally against the law. And everyone here knows it. I'm going to have to turn these people in. Now you. That's different. By law, I don't have to turn in a family member. How they got that on the statutes I don't know. But you can come with me. I probably can even get you your job back. If you agree to be debriefed."

"Yeah, how many medicines will they use on me to bring me into compliance, I wonder? Thanks, but I'll take my chances with this group. Gail, come on, if you were real sick, I'd do anything to help you. Right now, we've got a police officer's son. His family resources are fully used. He's only nine. What if you had a kid? What if we had a kid? Wouldn't we try anything to save him? Especially if he could be saved, and the only thing stopping the doctors was some bureaucrat." John quickly added, "No offense. Think, Gail. For once in your life, think for yourself. Don't you see? You could need a place like this some day. I could need a place like this. We're going to get old at the very least. I've seen what the government offers. It's not what I want."

"Save it, John." Gail said forcefully. "You think I haven't heard all this. Be a grown up. Be realistic. It's a small planet. We have to share. I'm sorry about the little boy, but there are other little boys getting care whose families maybe haven't overused or abused the system.

Maybe they were smart and saved their allotment. I'm not throwing away my career for your weak arguments. I want you back. I really do. But you don't seem to want to come back, do you?"

John was quiet. Then, "It's tempting. Life was easier when I didn't have to worry about anything. I had you. I had the Wellness Center. I had my pills. I wish I could be content with that again. But I don't think I can. And I can't let you take away my new life. A life that means something to me. That I care about."

"What are you saying?" Gail said noticing that John stood between her and the door.

"Don't be scared; they aren't going to hurt you. I'm not going to hurt you. They are just going to watch you very carefully. Probably take your modem and computer. 'Til they can figure out what they are going to do. Since you won't help, I'm assuming you won't tell me what you have told your supervisor already. Knowing you, it could be you've told him everything. It could be you've told him nothing and are saving what you have learned for the big brass, so you can make a giant leap in your career."

"I'm telling you nothing, John. Nothing you can say will make me change my mind. So just go on, get out of here. There is nothing left for us to say to each other. It's over. You don't owe me a thing. And I certainly don't owe you anything."

"So this is it. This is how it ends. Can't you try to be just a little human for a change, Gail? Can't you see that people aren't robots or computers? They are complex and have feelings."

"That doesn't mean the government system is wrong." Gail set her chin stubbornly. "I can certainly get by without you. Really when I think back to our marriage, you just leaned on me back then. Used me really, John, you never really cared about me. I took care of you, if anything. You needed me. I don't need you, and I never did. So forget the old time's sake routine. It will get you nothing. Now go on. Leave me alone." With that Gail flopped down on the bed and turned her face away from John.

John searched his feelings. Nothing. He felt nothing for this woman. "Somehow, having you to lean on just doesn't tempt me at all to come back. Not at all. You can have your phony job, phony friends and phony life. I'll be staying right here where my life finally means something." With that, he left.

Gail immediately sat up and pensively chewed on her already well-worn right index finger.

To Rufuos, the hour Dr. Chambers spent examining his son, Aaron, seemed to stretch into days. Dr. Chambers had to help his boy. He just had to. There had to be an answer for Rufuos' nine-year-old son, a boy of delightful spirit and innocence. Rufuos had lost his own brother to this disease. It was rare but familial. He and his wife had even considered not having children at all, but then the new medicines were developed, and they naively had thought they had nothing to worry about.

Boy, were they wrong. Anymore, it didn't matter how far science had come. Without a way to get care, all the new innovations and discoveries would be of no help to the sick. This disease had been curable for years now. The medicines had not been available for his brother. But they existed now. It was just getting them that was so difficult. Rufuos' seven-year-old daughter had been treated for juvenile diabetes successfully, which was how the family's medical allotment had been depleted. Now they were telling him, Rufuos, a father, that his son could have no more of anything. A waiting period of two years had to be satisfied. This is the fair way, the lady at the The System Office had informed him. We must be fair.

"They must think we ordinary people are just plain dumb," Rufuos muttered to himself as he waited for Dr. Chambers to finish his examination of Aaron. Rufuos was well aware of the fact that those high-level government officials who needed healthcare and support received it no matter what their level of usage was. The System worked for them because they were exempted. There was a *special system of care* in place for them. Naturally they thought their lives were more important than the average person's. Where would they be without me and others like me? What reward was there for being a policeman on the street? If anyone deserved special consideration, it's those who stood on the front lines in the cities of this nation.

"The police protect your right to your elite rights," Rufuos thought angrily. "Who protects my boy? Me. I'm it for him. I'm his only chance." Rufuos stood up and began to pace. Is it worth the risk? His wife was worried, he knew. If he went to jail or worse happened to him, who would help her with the kids and house and everything? He understood how she felt. But how could he live with himself if he didn't fight for his boy?

Suddenly his phone vibrated. Sis. He had totally forgotten about her. His partner didn't even know where he was right now. He had told no one except his wife. No one was to know. Not even Sis. Especially not Sis. Sis came from all kinds of connections. Everyone figured police work for her was just a fun activity. Rufuos felt he knew better. Sis had a real fondness for the job. But he did believe that she would never be in a situation such as his. Her allotment would never be erased. Her connections to high-level government officials were always there to help her out. Still, he would have to respond to her sometime.

But not now, not yet. He had to know if he was in time for his boy. After he talked to Dr. Chambers. Then he would talk to Sis. But still he must not tell her everything. She might spill the information—not meaning to. And she might not approve. He couldn't be the one responsible for the wrong people finding out about St. Luke's. He couldn't be the one to get these people in trouble with the government. They had agreed to help his son. He couldn't betray them. These so called criminals.

# CHAPTER 19

The sign on the door to his office said: VICTOR SWAIN, HEAD OFFICER, FIELD OPERATION, MEDICAL RESEARCH REGULATIONS AND REQUIREMENTS. But Victor had always felt he really should be referred to as the Everything Man. When they want something, I get it for them. 'Course it had to be this way. The government had to survive. Those in power were needed and really were more important than the average citizen on the street. And when a high-level official needed his help, he provided it. His contribution made the System work. His discreet studies of illegal field hospitals kept him up to date. He knew that the outside or Underground as they immaturely liked to be called sometimes learned things that the Government Medical Distribution System didn't. This was understandable. They didn't have to follow rules.

The government knew where these Underground hospitals were and what they were doing. Poor simple minded Gail Tilden and others like her helped out with that. They didn't have the big picture. They just acted as unwitting informants and that worked for him. All of this remained unknown to most Americans. A secret kept in order to maintain stability of The U.S. Healthcare Distribution System that struggled under huge bureaucracy, high costs, and limited resources. As long as these field hospitals, as he liked to call them, did not procreate at too rapid a pace, as long as the average person stayed within the confines of the U.S. Government Healthcare System, we would all be OK. That way, when a highly placed official needed healthcare of a higher level of sophistication than that supplied by the government to ordinary Americans, the field hospital supplied an alternative. Doctors in those hospitals were able to experiment to some degree, so that really complicated medical problems could be solved, and people, like Senator Debra Jamison, whose office had just called, had additional recourse.

The senator might become President one day. Her health issues were a deeply guarded secret. Her visit to an outcountry Underground hospital likewise would be kept secret. Hopefully, she would be in and out in no time. This particular hospital had not been used heretofore. As customary, he had sent a mole, a physician, of course, to check out the place and give him regular updates on medical practices there. Naturally, after the senator had availed herself of the services there, St. Luke's would have to be terminated. How else could you keep something like this secret? He had no guilt about that. Another clinic would sprout up. They always did. Sometimes the government even supplied moles to help. The status quo. That was really the bottom line when it came to his job. Maintain the status quo and supply a way in for high-level officials who needed care. After all, the average citizens needed these same people to run the government. Health issues for them were of utmost priority. The average factory worker or farmer could be replaced. Not so in the cases of the government where talented and brilliant people kept the nation running smoothly.

Senator Debra Jamison from Pennsylvania had served on numerous Congressional Committees. Well-respected and well-liked by friend and foe alike, she managed to keep secret a disease she had battled the last three years. Her specialty was bank regulation, but she had done a little bit of everything. Now the Democratic Party had listed her as the most likely candidate for their party in the next presidential election still two years away. Her husband, Todd Hartman, a successful ACLU lawyer, supported her in her lofty goals. It was he who had called Victor this morning with the medical update on the senator. Victor knew the irony in all of this. The ACLU often made public their support of the U.S. Government Healthcare System. The Medical System was not going away. It would last. Places like St. Luke's were allowed to continue only until they were no longer useful for special needs that occasionally arose. Of course, Todd saw no conflict between getting his wife Underground care and supporting the U.S. Government Healthcare System for the average American.

Enough of his musings. Victor needed to contact the mole at St. Luke's to make sure the physician most capable of treating Debra's problems would be there. After his last communication from Gail Tilden, he had gotten the impression that something was not quite right there. He might have to find another site for the senator. Maybe his mole would be more helpful than that novice, Tilden. He used a secure line to make the call.

Debra sat down in front of the lighted mirror on her vanity. Her face was changing rapidly. She could see that for herself. Her limp black hair, once full and wavy, now framed a colorless face. Large dark circles negated her once beautiful green eyes. She looked as if the aging process had accelerated into high gear. No one wanted an old looking president. At fifty-eight she was hardly old. On the outside, the signs of wear and tear from her disease were definitely there. The disease had bounded through every organ of her body. At the rate she was aging, she would soon be retired in a nursing care facility. No one would trust her intellectual ability. Even Todd, loyal Todd, would lose interest, she feared. She believed he had been loyal so far, but how long could that last if his wife looked ancient? Calling Victor had been Todd's idea. A surprise to her because she would have thought that he would be philosophically opposed to such an idea. Becoming desperate, Debra didn't seem to have any scruples left. She only wanted to live. And by that she meant live fully. All her life she had planned and organized her actions, always with the goal of becoming president some day. Now, things were looking good for her. All she had to do was stay healthy, and she would definitely have a chance at being the president of this nation. She knew she would be an able leader for this country.

But first her health. She had to get that turned around. She had to find a way to improve her chances for a full recovery. Debra was enough of a pragmatist to use whatever resources were available to get her health back on track. She trusted Victor. He had an excellent reputation for being capable and discreet. Two very unusual qualities in these times. Actually, she was looking forward to getting out of Washington for a while. It would be an adventure. A fruitful one she hoped.

At that very moment her husband was meeting with Victor to secure a hospital location for her.

"How will you reach this doctor? Without giving yourself away, I mean," Todd Hartman asked.

"That's my job. Let me worry about it," Victor replied. "I have experience with this. I'm sure the physician will call me back. The doctor can't always get away or be alone. I'm sure we'll make contact before the day is through."

"I hope they can help." Todd Hartman paced back and forth in Victor's office. "How can we trust these people to work on my wife?"

"Oh, you don't have to worry about that. She'll get the finest care."

"But aren't they angry with the government? Having to set up outside the government? You know what I mean?"

"I do know what you mean. But you really don't have to worry. They are quite altruistic actually. As long as they feel their operation is safe, they will not care who Debra is."

"How do we know they will keep all this a secret? How can we avoid leaks?"

"That, too, I will handle. You have nothing to worry about. It's all going to be fine. Debra will be fine. She'll be the next president. You'll see. No one will know about St. Luke's. We keep a tight control on these places. They won't dare to release information about her. It will all be fine. Especially for Debra. She just needs to plan her acceptance speech."

The phone rang. "There's my call. Please excuse me." He nodded to Hartman indicating their meeting had ended. Hartman hesitated as Victor turned his attention to his phone conversation. "Hello. Yes, it's a blood disorder." He paused. "I'm hoping you have someone there well-versed in the best medicines and latest techniques. You do? Sounds good. We'll arrange to move her in the usual way. She'll be there tonight. We expect the best."

He looked up. Todd still stood at the door. Victor just stared. Finally, Todd reluctantly left closing the door behind him.

Victor returned to his phone call, "Yes, I sent you another agent." Victor listened for a moment. "What happened? That's just her lack of experience and too much passion for her job. I'll speak to her on my next call. No, we won't be pulling her. She has to stay. She serves as a good diversion. That way they won't be looking for you. We need her there. What? Her husband? What is he doing there? It's OK. Don't worry." He paused. "Look, if they're worried about her, that should make your job easier. We just want the place to stay open long enough for our patient to gain treatment. Then, we'll get you out of there and plant you someplace else. So sit tight and don't worry. We're going to come in and get you in the near future."

After a night of tossing and turning, it was almost a relief to get out of bed and face another day. Or so Gail Tilden thought until she realized she was still stuck out here in the middle of nowhere. This was one ridiculous place. No wonder John fits in here perfectly. She smiled at the thought. She would play along and watch for a chance to escape even though her government supervisor had told her to stay put. What did he know? He wasn't here to experience this nonsense. Yesterday, she had been looking out her dorm window in boredom only to spy that police officer she had met in Baltimore. What was he doing here? She couldn't tell.

He had pulled his car around away from view. She suspected that he was here undercover. When her supervisor had called last night, she had begun thinking that maybe the government had sent in this police officer to help in the takeover. That idea really made her tense and angry. Why did they think she couldn't take care of this on her own? She didn't need help from the outside.

There was a soft knock on the door.

"Who is there?" she asked.

"It's John."

"Go away. We have nothing to talk about"

"Thought you might like some breakfast? A walk outside? Aren't you sick of being in this room?"

"Oh all right," this after a big sigh. "Just a minute. Let me put some clothes on." She slipped into a pair of jeans and white turtleneck sweater and then swung the door open. "What do you suggest for today's entertainment?" she said sarcastically.

"Thought you'd like to meet out newest patient."

"I don't think so."

"Come anyway. You might learn something." Her interest picked up. He was right. Never knew what you might see. She might see something John didn't even want her to know about.

"Oh, OK, I'm coming." She swung the door open. He stood, hands in his khaki pants pockets. She looked up at him, "You look … relaxed."

"Hmmm. Yes, I guess I am. This place agrees with me."

He smiled down at her.

"I still say you are making a mistake."

"Oh, maybe. But I'll take my chances."

"Don't go thinking you're better than me. 'Cause you are most definitely not."

He laughed. "There's my Gail Tilden. Superior attitude. Darlin' did I ever have a chance competing with you?"

"Who are you?"

He just laughed again in answer. "Oh, OK, I'll stop acting happy. I know how that annoys you."

She followed him down the stairs, out to the courtyard and over to the main building. Inside she continued to follow John through the maze that she still marveled at. How they found their way around was beyond her. But it wasn't long before John stopped at one of the patient's rooms. He poked his head in and said good morning to the patient inside.

"Would you like some company?"

"Sure," came the sound of a small voice from inside the room.

"This is Ms. Tilden. Ms. Tilden, this is Aaron."

"Hello Aaron," Gail said. Gail came forward tentatively.

"Aaron is here for a while, while the doctors check him out. Then home he will go, back to the city. Though we would like to keep him because he is a great joke teller. Go ahead, Aaron, tell this lady a joke."

Aaron smiled shyly at Gail. "What do you call a sheep with no legs?"

"I don't know. Tell me," Gail smiled.

"A cloud!" Aaron said. He giggled that beautiful innocent giggle that all children start out with but usually have lost by the time they are Aaron's age.

"Can I tell you another?"

After the third one, Gail pulled up a chair. "I think this is going to take a while." She smiled and sat down.

Dr. Chambers stuck his head in the room at one point and asked John to come help him with another patient. John was reluctant to leave his charge.

He looked at Gail, "You OK here?"

"Sure," she said not looking at him.

"How about you, sport?" John reached over and tousled Aaron's soft black curly hair.

"I'm OK, I'm almost ten."

"Oh right, you are getting old, Aaron." John gave him one more smile and left without looking at Gail.

But when he got with Dr. Chambers alone, he expressed his concerns. Chambers replied, "Where is she going to run off to? There is nothing for miles around."

"You're right. She doesn't have any survival skills."

Chambers glanced back into the room, "Who knows? Maybe we can win her over to our side just by being nice. What do you think?"

John thought a minute. He looked at Chambers. They both laughed.

"Nah, won't happen," John said.

"Right. People don't change that much. Or that fast. Except for you, John."

He had changed. Was it that he was no longer on his meds? Or was it because he actually took care of people now? In response to Chambers, he could only say, "I guess I have."

John looked back toward the room they had just left, "If her boss told her to think differently, then she could change. But she doesn't have an original thought in her brain. It's all been force fed to her over the years." He then turned his attention to their next patient. "Let's check on Mr. Miller."

"OK, but first tell me, are you sure you are the same guy Marcie and I picked up alongside the road? I mean, maybe you are the one human being who can change."

John stopped, looked at him and smiled, "I haven't changed. I just couldn't be myself before. This is really me." Then as he entered the next patient's room, "Hello, Mr. Miller. How are you doing today? Need any more pain meds? I brought Dr. Chambers. He'll fix you up."

McClaren worried tirelessly through the week to get his sermon just right for Sunday morning. One might wonder why he went to so much trouble for the group of less than ten who gathered at St. Luke's on Sunday morning. McClaren had a ready answer for that one. He viewed his whole experience here at St. Luke's as a special test. After all, Abraham was tested. Job was tested. Jesus himself was tested. This was McClaren's test. And he intended to pass this test with flying colors. Determined that even if only one person attended Sunday service, that person would understand that he or she was important to him, McClaren, and, by extrapolation, to God.

Further, McClaren was convinced that even if the doctors, nurses, and techs seemed untouched by his efforts, there might be one or two who admired what he was doing. They might even think something good might come out of all of this. He hoped so. He thought his sermons were pretty good. He wasn't being conceited. He just felt they were pretty good. He worked plenty hard on them. Suddenly the doorbell interrupted, and McClaren pulled himself away from his musings.

He headed for the front door, checked the peephole and saw a man with a black cap standing on his front porch. Looked official. The butterflies in McClaren's stomach began to bounce around. He took a deep breath and opened the door.

"Reverend McClaren?"

"Yes?"

"I'm a driver for Ms., I mean the Honorable Debra Jamison. She has come here to see you."

"Really?"

"Yes," said a beautiful deep voice. The senator had followed her driver to the porch. "I would very much like to talk to you, Reverend McClaren."

There was a beautiful, mature woman to go with the voice. But McClaren noticed the sad green eyes first.

"Good morning. I'm Debra Jamison. Perhaps you have heard of me?" She saw question and doubt cross the reverend's face. "Perhaps not. It doesn't matter. I'm hoping you can help me. May we come in?"

"Of course! I'm forgetting my manners. Certainly come in. How can I be of service to you?" McClaren led both the driver and Debra into the sanctuary of St. Luke's.

"Well, quite simply I'm in need of medical care. I hear you can help me." Debra looked directly at McClaren.

"Don't really know to what you are referring,"

"Are you Reverend McClaren?"

"Yes."

"And this is St. Luke's?"

"Definitely."

"And I am in outcountry," she paused and gazed out the large church window, "for the first time in a very long time?"

"Oh, yes ma'am. No doubt about that."

"Well, then, I think you can help me. You see. I may not look it. But I am very sick. Very sick. I cannot stress that enough. I've tried many doctors and health advisors. But still no improvement. I have heard you might be able to help. I thought it was true that your people never push the suffering aside. Am I right about that or am I wrong?"

McClaren studied his liver spotted hands for a while and then said, "We don't know you."

"You can check me out. I'm sure you will discover that I am as sick as I am saying that I am. Now, you have at your disposal people who can help me. And may I say that I am in a position to help you? Are you not interested in changing the government's form of health-care delivery?"

"I don't know," McClaren said noncommittally. "Do you think it needs changing?"

Debra smiled slightly, "You sound like one of my colleagues." She breathed deeply. "You help me, and I may be able to help you. You know, I could be president some day—if your people are able to help me with my illness. Now what do you say?"

"Could you excuse me for a moment?"

"Certainly. Take your time. You understand I need to sit down. We'll wait in the car."

McClaren looked at the senator, "You are welcome to sit here in the sanctuary." He looked at her driver. "Both of you. I won't be long."

# Chapter 20

Marilyn tried to hide her feelings, but the thought of Senator Debra Jamison becoming a patient at St. Luke's incensed her.

"Let her use the Wellness Center in her area," was Marilyn's response when McClaren informed her of their latest guest.

"This sure is gettin' to be an active place," McClaren said. He had corralled Marilyn along with Chambers, John and a few of the other doctors and techs into his cramped office. "We can't leave them out there in the sanctuary forever. My absence has to be making them more convinced that they are in the right place."

It was John who spoke up, "Let's let them in. They are going to report us no matter what. So at least we keep them here. Maybe we'll get protection. Should we talk to Marcie and Salmund about this?"

"No," replied McClaren, "I think I want to get them out now without any knowledge of this. They'll be safer that way. Don't want them seen by these two, so I'll send them back to the city. I think they will agree with my judgment on this. As for our new guests, let's do as John suggests and let them in." McClaren headed for the door. He turned back to Chambers, "We'll leave it to you doctors to decide if the senator is truly ill." He then turned to look at John. "John, I think maybe you are the one to show them in."

John looked up, startled, shrugged his shoulders and said, "Sure, fine."

"Yes, come with me."

McClaren and John found Debra and her driver right where McClaren had left them, "So, Senator Jamison, we've decided to accept you as a patient. Of course, we expect your driver to stay as well."

Senator Jamison smiled and nodded, "I expected he would be included." She turned to her driver, "Charles, please bring our things. We're staying."

"Charles, I'll go with you." McClaren turned to Debra, "John, here, will show you to your room." He and Charles left them. Debra looked at John.

"Hmmm. You don't look like a criminal." John didn't answer. Debra held her hand and they shook hands. "Are you going to be my doctor?"

John said, "No, I think Dr. Chambers will be taking care of you. I'm just a tech here."

"Really? I thought you were a doctor. Where did you get your training? Or, pardon me, I don't want to offend, maybe I should ask did you have any training?"

"Actually, I was trained at the University of Maryland Technical Training School."

"Really?"

"Yes." John couldn't help but feel friendly toward this lady. He liked her calmness. And she seemed genuinely interested in him. "I thought I knew quite a bit until I came here. But here they let me learn new stuff. Stuff they wouldn't allow me to do in the government system." He paused and looking directly at her, "No offense."

She laughed a full throaty laugh, "None taken. I like to think I can be a grownup in situations such as this." She took a long look around the sanctuary, "So, this is what a church looks like. I haven't traveled much, always going to school, and then working, and then the Senate."

John followed her gaze to the cross hanging behind the pulpit. Long shadows fell across the pews this late in the day.

On impulse, he asked her, "Are you a believer?"

"No," she responded quietly. "Must one convert to be accepted here?"

"Of course not," he replied. "All are welcome here, even some who would want to destroy us."

"Meaning me?"

"Among others."

"I have no intention of harming any of you."

"Perhaps not. But others know you are here."

"I could have used an alias."

"Yes."

"But I didn't. Even though others wanted me to. I refused to be deceptive with Reverend McClaren or any of you."

"Why are you here?"

"Why? Because I am very sick."

"Why didn't you go to a U.S. System Hospital?"

Debra didn't say anything.

"Right. You are Debra Jamison, aren't you?"

"Yes."

"The same Debra Jamison who sits on the committee making decisions about how the Wellness Centers should be run?"

"I have been on that committee. Yes."

"Exactly, so tell me again why you are here."

Debra said nothing. Just stared back.

John smirked. "Senator, you may have good intentions. You may even applaud what we do here. But I believe later you will deny you were ever here. Right now you have something to gain by being here, and that is the best medical care. Something apparently you did not believe you could get from your U.S. Government Wellness Centers. You didn't ask why I am here, did you?"

He waited for an answer, but got none. He breathed. "OK, follow me. Let's go downstairs to the dungeon of illegal medical activity." Debra Jamison followed him as he led her into the hospital.

"Is he in?" Paul leaned over her desk to get Melody (Matthew Salmund's secretary) to respond.

She looked up briefly from her computer and said, "Go on in. He always has time for you."

"Thanks." Melody watched as Paul strode briskly into Matthew's office and heard him say, "Matthew, we've got a problem." Normally, Melody would have found eavesdropping a good way to fill the next hour, but her online soap had an interesting plotline happening, which she wanted to catch. So she turned her attention back to her screen.

Matthew knew from experience not to worry too much when Paul acted crazed as he did right now. "Sit down, Paul, and let's hear about this problem."

"It's St. Luke's."

"What about it?"

"Did you know their patient population includes now one senator, one son of a police officer, regular visits by the cop, at least one government agent who constantly converses with Victor Swain, not to mention correspondence between the aforementioned senator and her spouse? We know from hacking away at communications that at least one doctor feeds information to Victor. That's known information, Matthew. I think we gotta think about pulling the plug—getting everyone out of there and relocated."

"How will we accomplish this, Paul?"

"Is Marcie still out there?"

"Actually no, but I can always contact her. She watches her communication extremely carefully, as you know." Matt leaned back in his chair and smiled as he thought of Marcie.

"Come on, Matt, we need a decision. Soon. Real soon."

"I don't know if we should proceed too fast here, Paul. After all, we've got the Honorable Debra Jamison visiting. Wouldn't want to cut that visit short. She could help our cause."

"Help us?! Do you know who her husband is?" Paul asked.

"Of course I know. I know as well as you Todd Hartman basically runs the ACLU. He, like the rest of his ilk, wants the same healthcare for everyone except for the people he loves. Right now, I don't think he wants anything bad to happen at St. Luke's just the same as us. At least not while Debra remains. After, well, that will be different. Meanwhile, I want the doctors to take excellent care of her like they do with all of their patients. We'll figure this out. I agree that it's a problem, Paul. But let's not panic just yet. That's how we make mistakes. Carefully. That's the way to do it."

Paul frowned.

Matt groaned, "OK, what else?"

"I'm just thinking. What if we have to hold her there? Remember, these are doctors and nurses plus one minister. Don't know if they can handle that."

"They'll be fine. The place is remote. There is no place for her to run to and besides, they're already managing with Ms. Tilden.

"So, how many kids do you have, Ms. Tilden?" Aaron asked politely. He liked this new lady; she was pretty and smelled nice. He would rather have been playing the latest piloting mission game on his computer with his best friend, James, but this lady would have to do for now. And for a long time maybe. His daddy had said he might have to stay here a while. It was fun at first, but after several weeks had gone by, Aaron missed everybody from his home complex."

Ms. Tilden smiled, "I don't have any."

"None?"

"Not a single one. What do you think of that?"

"Are you married?"

Good question. "Yes, I am."

"Are you sick then, like my mom's friend, Ashleigh? She can't have babies because she is sick inside."

"No, it's not that either. I just never thought I would be a good mommy, I guess."

"Oh, I think you would. My mom says babies are the most fun. I don't know for sure about that. When my sister Karyn gets to crying big time, my mom doesn't seem to like it so much."

"I'm sure she doesn't," Gail smiled.

"Is it true that we are illegal here?" Aaron changed the subject abruptly. "Is it true we could go to jail? My dad says it don't matter for me 'cause they wouldn't really put me in jail. And I overheard him say to Mama that if I don't go here, then I'm out of luck, but he used a bad word with it and my mama started to cry and that's how come my daddy is doing something that's not legal. I wouldn't be afraid to go to jail instead of my daddy, no sir. But he keeps telling me that's no problem, no sir, not as long as that senator lady is here. We'll be just fine, just fine staying here and lettin' the doctors take care of me."

"I'm sure you will be. Let's leave some of this to the grownups, shall we? Even though I can see you are extremely smart and probably could take care of things better than us grownups."

"Are you afraid to go to jail?"

"Oh, I would be afraid, but I don't expect that to happen. I'm here to observe and I have permission."

"Permission, really?"

"Yep, it's all clear for me."

"I feel bad sometimes though because, Ms. Tilden, what if there is some kid just my age who is just as sick as me who needs Dr. Chambers? We don't have permission to be here like you do."

Gail just nodded.

"How come my daddy couldn't get permission for me?"

Gail didn't know what to say. "You know, I think I am needed in the computer room right about now. We'll talk about this more the next time I visit."

"OK," Aaron said, "you would have been a great mama. Not like that Marcie lady. She is so mean."

"I don't know about that. She is nice too, I'm sure." Gail said.

So now, of course, sleep wouldn't come. Gail tossed and turned. Got up, had some water. Changed position. Counted back from 400. Nothing worked. And she didn't want to face it. No sir, as Aaron would say. She didn't want to face the fact that a nine year-old boy's talk would keep her up. She was a grownup, wasn't she? Guess not, her inner voice responded. She got up for the zillionth time, washed her face and went back to bed. But sleep never did really come. She never totally let go.

"Gail, you in there?" Gail sat up abruptly. Morning had come. Finally. She had drifted off to light sleep just as the sun came up. "Wake up Gail. They want you down there." Another loud knocking.

"OK, OK, stop banging on the door! I'm coming." She dragged herself out of bed and opened the door. Disheveled and panting, John stood before her. "They've called a meeting. Want you there. I don't know why. In fact, I might as well tell you I told them to leave you out. But McClaren would have none of it. So get dressed fast and come on."

"And what if I don't?" Gail decided to be coy.

"Don't give me that. You're dying to know what it's about. You always want to be in the inner circle. You know that. Here's your chance. Get dressed. I'll wait. Out here."

She wanted to slam the door in his face. But instead, he reached in and pulled the door closed firmly. What to wear? She grabbed her navy business suit and stuck a pocket size recorder with a fresh flash in her jacket pocket.

The sanctuary lights were turned up high. But still it felt creepy to Gail as she joined the others. The entire staff had seated themselves in groupings of two's and three's. McClaren made the announcement that a nurse and a doctor and one tech remained downstairs with the patients. John and Gail came in from the back. Gail seated herself just behind a group of doctors. John went over and joined Dr. Chambers.

"So glad you could make it, Ms. Tilden."

Gail nodded at the minister, and looked around at the others. A number of faces had turned, and Gail was taken off guard when she saw Rufuos frowning at her. What was he doing here she wondered. Then she realized that it was his son, Aaron, she had been visiting. The Aaron whose words kept her up at night. So a police officer, a man of the law, had his son here in outcountry as a patient. This would spice up her report a bit.

"Here's the thing." McClaren began talking. Everyone stopped their various conversations and looked up to the front of the church where McClaren stood. "Paul came on board recently. You all know him by now. You also know he established a computer security system for us which works quite nicely. We have reached the point, thanks to Paul, where we can obtain information without being tracked. An unusual feat to be sure. We owe you, Paul, a huge debt of gratitude. We have now the advantage of anticipating government activity. A lucky thing for us. Up to now, we have been ignored. They know, of course, we are here. After all, how else would Senator Debra Jamison have found us?"

Senator Jamison? Gail sat up suddenly. What was she doing here? And why hadn't her supervisor told her? Gail looked over at John instinctively who she discovered returned a smug smile. She obliged with a smirk of her own in an attempt to cover her embarrassment at not being included in the loop of information. Stunned, she realized that if she didn't know, that meant another government agent was inside. Someone else had been providing information to the government. She looked back at John and saw again that he returned her gaze. Gail saw from his thoughtful expression that he, too, had come to the same conclusion as she.

Simultaneously, they scanned the gathering trying to discern who that person was. They had no clue. No one had appeared suspicious. Gail had only viewed these people as dedicated medical professionals. In fact, she had concluded that they would not be good at any other area, especially not spying.

John's mind performed similar scanning and sifting functions. Who could it be? His wife appeared totally flummoxed, and he almost felt sorry for her. She could only view the fact that she had been ignored as a total professional insult. And since her only identity came from her work, that could be monumental in her mind.

The mole sat back comfortably in the pew, eyes on whoever spoke, trying to appear professional but relaxed, so no one would suspect. Gail would be searching the group for a likely suspect. Government field agents were extremely competitive by nature. Gail was no exception. The mole's eyes stayed first on McClaren, and then on Paul, who had been speaking.

"So as Reverend McClaren said, we have a very good security program in place. We also have excellent hacking capabilities. That is what I do. We also have been more free to communicate with other non-government medical facilities, and we have learned some disturbing news. News that we felt you all should be privy to. Before I speak to that, I want to say that you are all probably concerned about Ms. Tilden's presence here at this meeting. I believe you will understand why as I reveal the information we have learned. It will affect all of us, even Ms. Tilden."

"Several other medical facilities," Paul continued, "across this nation have informed us that we have made a fatal mistake in admitting a senator. We, here at St. Luke's, mistakenly thought that having a senator as a patient might perhaps influence our government in the direction we want it to take in providing thorough medical care to the American people. Unfortunately for us, and too late for us, the real situation is that the government has a policy." Paul paused and looked down for a second, "a policy of destroying the facility once the public person has been discharged." He looked out at the faces of the medical care providers at St. Luke's, and said quietly. "I'm so sorry."

Reverend McClaren immediately rose from his seat, patted Paul on the back and indicated to him that he should return to his seat. "Now friends, we must not panic. We need to have some time to think this through. To decide the proper course of action for us. We thank you, Paul, for helping us. And your warning may save us. We hope. We hope. OK. I think we all know we can handle transferring our operation somewhere else. But it will take quite a bit of planning and work. So, we will need to keep Ms. Jamison here as long as necessary to get that plan in order. I know none of you signed on to be jailers, but the fact is that she is our protection. Her presence here will keep the patients safe as well."

"This stinks," John said. His blood boiled. He had finally found a place in life that worked for him. And now the thought that this could end incensed him.

And then there was Gail. He realized he felt nothing for her.

"John, can't hear you. What did you say?"

John stood up. "I said this stinks. Why can't they leave us alone? We aren't doing anything wrong."

"Please don't get upset, John. Actually we are all upset. We know that the work we do here is good. And obviously some in Congress and the rest of the government do also. But we must be realistic."

"What are they going to do? They can't tell us to leave."

"They will tell us. And if we don't comply, they will make us."

"Can't we just leave for a bit and then come back?"

"No," Gail said quietly. She looked directly at John and then the others, "No, they will destroy everything. You, the hospital, every-thing. Even me, if I am still here." Her voice trailed away and she sat.

John saw her now as a stranger. Did he actually ever live with Gail? Did he ever really know her? He probably should hate her now, but all he could feel was pity. He sat down, overcome with sadness.

"Ms. Tilden is telling the truth," Reverend McClaren said. "I have not really been graphic in my description of how these other facilities ceased functioning. Much suffering and death occurred. We're talking tanks and bombs. Destruction like you haven't seen in a very long time. It's all very well and good and noble to die for a cause, but no one in the city will know of it. No one will care that we have died. And those people who need us—they will be the ones who will suffer the most. They will have trouble finding another source of care. We need to formulate a plan. We need time to do that. If we decide to pack up and go, we need time for that too. We even need time to de-cide to stay and die. I, for one, will not allow the patients to stay under such circumstances."

McClaren took a breath and then continued, "I am going to spend the next few days in conference with some other locations. Paul will be working his computer as usual. The rest of you are to go on as if this meeting had not occurred. Dr. Chambers will continue to treat Senator Jamison. I must also add that the situation is not to be discussed within the hearing of the patients. We want to be able to present a plan to them when we tell them. Their situation is our number one priority as always."

The meeting over, Paul purposefully strode into his computer office. He stopped short when he found Marcie sitting in his chair.

"What are you doing here?" Paul asked.

"Just checking in. I used your surveillance equipment to listen in on Reverend McClaren's meeting. I have only one question. Why are you going so slowly? I think we should move everyone and every piece of medical equipment out now while we have the chance. Anything not essential to the care of the current residents can be left here."

"It takes time to figure out where we are going, you know, Marcie."

"Always excuses." Marcie replied. "We need to get out now while we can still go and go silently."

Paul sat down opposite Marcie in the only extra chair in the cramped office. "We have reasons." Paul said. "Trust us a little bit won't you, Marcie?"

"You know, Paul, I've worked hard for our cause and more than once I've been out there on my own—no one to help me should I need it. Now you want me to risk my life by hanging out here when the government is waiting, just waiting, to take you and this whole place out. Don't think I'm ready to give up that much for your cause. Besides it's not practical. I'm too good at what I do for you to lose me."

"Oh don't go dramatic on me, Marcie, it doesn't become you. You've made a nice cozy living in the procurement business. I bet your holdings are at banks all over the world." Marcie squirmed just a bit and averted her eyes. "You think we don't know how you operate Marcie? We know you like to stash your earnings away. And we know you have no special motivation except to make money."

"Oh, please. We all know about you, Matt, and Christiane. You've turned this into some holy exercise. It's time you both grew up. Bad things happen. Christiane was real unlucky, but to devote your whole life to avenging the poor treatment she received, that's just plain silly. How can you help anyone when your mind is stuck in the past? Now back to the day at hand and our imminent destruction. What is to be done about it?"

"Funny you should be so adamant about the whole business, Marcie. We're sure you want to save yourself and maybe a few others. After all, if we're not here, you have no job. Isn't that right?"

"What are you saying?" Marcie began to feel nervous. What was he getting at?

"Well, I'm saying that there are many ears around—ears that will carry information back to the government. And we sure don't want that, do we Marcie? No, we don't want that."

"What are you leading up to, Paul?"

"We're on the lookout for a mole in our operation. If we announce to the community what our plans are, the government is going to receive that information immediately. Something we don't want. We want to retain just a day or two of time."

Marcie thought about this. "Who do you suspect?"

Paul dropped his eyes to the stack of reports in his lap.

"Oh, no!"

"Oh, yes."

"Oh, no, you aren't really thinking?"

"Oh, it definitely came up."

"No! You and Matt couldn't possibly believe that."

"Oh, yeah, we could. We are suspicious. Of everyone."

"But me?" Marcie's voice grew, but quickly she regained her composure. Why did she feel so hurt? "Me, come on now, Paul, you know that just cannot be. I've been loyal. You know that, Paul. And Matt knows as well. It isn't me. Wait'll I see him again."

"I have to be sure before I show my cards."

"You guys are losing it if you think I would side with the lousy government on anything." Marcie rose and slammed her hands loudly down on the desk (Paul's desk actually). "I would never side with them," she yelled, now decisively. "Never! Don't you know that by now? Never ever. So just forget it."

"Well, it's someone. We know that, even if it's not you," Paul couldn't resist needling her just a bit, and he wanted to make sure she wasn't holding out on him. "We need to know who it is before we proceed. Can you at least see that? Do you see it, Marcie?"

Subdued, Marcie sat back down. "Yes, I see it, Paul. Don't know how you are going to figure this one out. But please don't waste any more of your time wondering about me. It ain't me. Just ain't so. Got it?"

"I know a way you could convince me. And everyone else."

She looked at him. "What? NO! Come on, I don't have a clue."

"Yeah, but you have certain observation skills, Marcie. Certain abilities not everyone has."

"You mean I'll roll with the slime if I have to."

"Yeah, that's exactly what I mean. You can do this. It can be your ultimate contribution."

"Yeah, but I don't want to make a contribution. I want to survive. That's it for me. And it's damn plenty enough."

"Come on, you know you can help us, and it won't even be that hard for you. Aren't you just a teensy bit bored right now?" Paul caught her eye, "Yeah, I thought so."

Marcie shrugged noncommittally.

"This will make life interesting for you again. So do I have an agreement?"

"Well, I don't know."

"Need an excuse? I'll pay you—a lot."

Marcie relaxed, "Deal."

Paul got up to leave. With his hand on the door he turned to Marcie and said, "I like to keep life simple."

# Chapter 21

Marcie watched from the hallway as Aaron entertained his visitor. Ms. Tilden did seem sincerely interested in what the boy was saying though Marcie cynically thought this behavior tied in perfectly with Ms. Tilden's act.

"Convincing, isn't she?" Startled by John's voice, Marcie turned to see him watching Gail as she had just been.

"She didn't want them, you know."

"What do you mean?" Marcie grabbed his arm and pulled him away from the door to Aaron's room. "Lower your voice." She whispered.

"I mean, kids. She didn't want kids. When we met, she said she did. But she lied. I'm just saying she is all an act."

Marcie stared at him.

"Right, I get it. You already know this. And I'm the idiot who didn't see it."

"Well, yeah."

He stood up taller and said, "I know who I have been. I am not going to be that person anymore."

"Really?"

"A person can change."

"Right."

"Whatever. Believe what you want."

"Why did you marry her?"

"I like taking care of people. She needed me when I met her. She was going nowhere with her career, and she didn't have any friends. Her parents were always, always on her case." He shook his head remembering how she had seemed then, so delicate, so pretty. "Her wickedness came out later. When she got the job with the U.S. Government Healthcare Distribution System, that's when she changed."

"Why did you stay with her? As you said, you don't have kids."

"Stupid, right? I know that now. I kept hoping she would change. And then I became the dependent one. The one who barely hung on. As I became weaker, she became stronger." He looked at Marcie. "Not everyone can be like you."

"What do you mean?"

"I mean you are unafraid. And you don't care what other people think. That's real power."

Marcie felt an uncharacteristic blush coming on. Embarrassed, she changed the subject.

"I've been staying away from your wife, but now I need to speak to her, to learn what she knows and doesn't know."

"Could you please just call her Gail? Please?"

She smiled. John thought she looked good when she smiled. Her hard face softened, but he said nothing.

"I think your, I mean, Ms. Tilden has been thrown a bit off by the fact that her bosses aren't telling her everything."

"Hmmm. That would definitely make her mad." He paused, took a breath and then said, "You don't really believe I would be on her side, do you?"

"Actually, I never really suspected you of that. I'm pretty good at assessing situations and people. So, no, I never thought that about you."

"But you think I'm weak."

"I don't know yet. I'm withholding judgment on that." She smiled again briefly, and John smiled back.

"You should smile more often."

"In my line of work there isn't much to smile about." She paused. Patted him on the arm, "I've got to get back to work. Ms. Tilden is next on my list."

"Right, OK," and John watched her walk toward Aaron's room.

Marcie stopped briefly at the door, looked back at John, and then went into Aaron's room.

"Hi, Aaron."

"Hi, Ms. Geck."

"Aaron, would you mind if I talked with Ms. Tilden for a while. I'll send her right back. I promise."

"Oh sure, it's OK," the boy replied, obviously disappointed with the interruption.

Ms. Tilden looked none too happy herself as she followed Marcie into the hallway. "What do you want?"

"Ms. Tilden, how would you like to redeem yourself? Be loved by everyone here at St. Luke's, including Aaron in there and Reverend McClaren. Maybe even get your slave boy, Macklin, back? What do you think?"

"You're disgusting."

"Yeah, well, right now you don't look so good to me. But that could change with just a bit of effort on your part."

"OK," Gail replied impatiently. "What do you want? Just tell me."

"Well, I want lots of things, but right now what I want most is some information from you. I'm sure even you have figured out that there is another agent here. Probably from the agency you report to. Maybe even from your boss. I would very much like to know who that person is."

Ms. Tilden shook her head laughing. "And tell me. Why should I help you? Why on earth and beyond would I want to do that?"

"Easy," Marcie grinned. She paused before saying, "You do want to live, don't you?"

"What are you talking about?"

"I'm talking about survival, Ms. Tilden. Something I pride myself at being very successful at. Something that is very important to me and should be to you."

"Look, I don't know what you are talking about, but I know of no such person here. I thought you'd be happy to know I was kept totally out of the loop."

"Well, normally, yes, I admit it, but we have a real problem here. Someone from the Government Healthcare Distribution System Compliance Department is here working and we need to find out who. 'Course I'll need you to keep mum about this, naturally."

"And why should I?"

"Again, you want to live. And somewhere in that cold heart of yours, you want Aaron and the other patients here to live."

"I think you're exaggerating this whole business. I haven't even been asked for a report yet."

"And didn't you wonder why? Your dear government, Ms. Tilden. They are coming to get us, and when the missiles start flying, do you think they are going to stop the operation just to save a certain

Ms. Tilden?" Marcie paused with her eyebrows raised, "Well, do you?"

"Even if I wanted to help you, what could I do? I don't know who this person might be."

"You need to start being—I know this will be difficult for you—sneaky when you report to your supervisor."

"I haven't been reporting to anyone since I have been here."

"Please don't waste my time with such ridiculous statements. Why in the world you thought you could have any kind of contact with the outside world without St. Luke's knowledge. Well, that's just the height of naiveté, Ms. Tilden, but then you really don't know much of the world, do you? Just what the government deems important for you, isn't that right? They control you, and, just for yucks, you control Macklin. Or used to. Pity that, Ms. Tilden."

So another night of tossing and turning for Gail Tilden. How had she gotten herself embroiled in such a mess? Life prior to her meeting with Chambers had been so orderly, so predictable and, most of all, so comfortable. She missed her friends, her sense of belonging which she used to get from her job. But no more. Now she realized that all the time she thought she was an appreciated employee, she was nothing to them. They didn't think highly enough of her to at least inform her that someone else was here. She determined that she would find out who. To that end, in her orderly way, Gail sat up in bed, turned on the bedside lamp, and began a list of suspects. Of course, she had to put every single person on the list who resided at St. Luke's with the exception of Aaron. She tried to make herself feel better by thinking that the additional agent had arrived because of Senator Jamison.

After completing the list, she decided to rank the people based on her own observations. Next to each name she put reasons. Like next to Macklin she put too weak, Chambers too nice, McClaren too strange, plus, she didn't think the government would ever approve of any cover that might encourage the return of religion. And so she continued through each name including Marcie's. She decided to ask her supervisor for info on Marcie as soon as the day began. Who cares who listens? The people here already know everything about me, so why restrain my conversations with the government?

"It's working," Paul said, as he watched the computer screen relay the intelligence he and Marcie had been waiting for. "She is talking to her supervisor about you, of all things. He looked at Marcie with appreciative eyes. You must have gotten to her."

Marcie smiled. "She is not a mystery to me. If we're lucky, she'll do the work for us. I'll check her room out today when she goes to see Aaron. Don't know what the deal is there, but she always keeps her appointment with him."

# CHAPTER 22

Rufuos couldn't shake the dream he had had this morning. It must have been around five a.m. In it, he wandered aimlessly around on foot. He kept wiping his sweating brow with the blue sleeve of his uniform. And stumbling. He looked down at his feet and saw rubble everywhere (where the pavement of the road used to be) so that gaining a decent footing was impossible. He couldn't get his bearings although he knew this was where he lived. But every building was black instead of the white concrete he knew it to be. Strangely, even while dreaming, his thought process told him that he would be cold when he awoke; therefore, he put his navy work sweater over his uniform making him too warm now. He ran to the old lady Marm's front door and pressed the buzzer but instead of lady Marm in her usual housecoat and hair net, there was a man. A big man, bigger than Rufuos who stood 6'2" in his stocking feet. Did he have shoes on? He couldn't see the man's feet. He looked down and the body of the man seemed to disappear in to the shadows. He looked up. There they were. The black eyes of evil. Rufuos couldn't release himself from the stare of those eyes. Eyes of evil. And then, even though he knew he should remember what the man was going to say, he never could. Even though it was always the same. Words were said before Rufuos could even ask the question. "Where's Aaron?" Thankfully, the alarm had wakened him, and he had somehow dressed and gotten to work still shaken by the images of his dream.

The phone at his right hand rang bringing Rufuos out of his dark musings. "OK, guess Monday had to start sometime," Rufuos said to himself as he snapped back to the reality of the squad room.

It was the lobby security officer.

"Officer King, we have someone who needs some help down here."

"Yeah, of course you do."

"We have a lady here, young lady who lost her baby. Needs help finding her baby. Do you want the case, or should I give it to someone else?"

"No, that's OK," Rufuos answered. "I'll take it. Might as well let the day begin. Gotta do something to earn my pay. Do you trust her on her own or should I come down and get her?"

"Nah, I think she is OK. Just upset is all. I'll send her up."

Rufuos hung up the phone. He shook himself in an effort to rid himself of the memory of his early morning nightmare. At least this would take his mind off of things. He caught Sis' eye at her desk. "We have a client coming up. Are you ready for the week to begin?"

"Sure," Sis replied, tossing back her perfectly cut blonde hair. "Bring it on. I'm ready." She grabbed her cup of already cold coffee and came over to his desk. "Had a great weekend," she said energetically. "How about you?"

"Oh yeah, the weekend was great. Stacey and I took the kids to the park for a picnic," Rufuos lied. Sis didn't need to know about Aaron. She might not understand.

Soon the elevator located across the room opened. A timid, poorly dressed, young woman hesitantly stepped off and looked furtively around the room. Her bedraggled honey brown long hair framed a pale face with round light hazel eyes. No one seemed to have noticed her entrance except for Sis and Rufuos who waved for her to come over. As she walked closer, they could tell she had been crying. Her full lips quivered as she approached the officers.

"I'm sorry to bother you, officers. I didn't know where else to go. I just didn't know," at which point she sank into the folding chair proffered by Rufuos and began sobbing, her head bent over her lap and held in her hands.

In between sobs, she stammered out, "My baby, my baby is lost. And it's totally my fault. I killed her. You might as well lock me up. It won't matter because I don't have a life if I don't have Lily."

"Lily's your baby?" Rufuos asked gently.

The woman looked up tears glistening in her round eyes. "Yes, Lily is my baby, my beautiful sweet baby."

"OK, Ms., uh, Ms.?"

"St. Clair. Sharon St. Clair. I never should have done what I did, Officer." She looked directly into Rufuos' eyes. The evil eyes of his morning terror flashed in front of him, and he realized he saw the exact opposite in this young woman's eyes. "I should have taken better care of her, so she wouldn't get sick," she continued. "It was my fault she got sick. My fault she is gone now." She began to lose control of her emotions once again. At which point Rufuos arose and went to get Ms. St. Clair some water.

After filling a cup at the water cooler, Rufuos turned and looked across the room at Ms. St. Clair and Sis. They were apparently deep in conversation, and Rufuos decided to wander into the coffee lounge for a few minutes to get himself some coffee, but mainly to allow Sis time to gather information from the young mother. People liked to talk to Sis. She had that quality. People would open up to her and tell her everything. Things they wouldn't tell their own mother. Rufuos not infrequently took advantage of that quality as he was doing now. He took his time fixing his coffee with a gigantic amount of cream and four sugars. He needed something to keep him going.

By the time he had returned, Sis was sitting at his desk typing up Ms. St. Clair's statement, and Ms. St. Clair had ceased crying.

"Well, OK, Ms. St. Clair, I'm glad you have pulled yourself together. Now I'm guessing you and Officer Leland have had a chance to get acquainted."

"Oh yes, she is wonderful. So understanding. I really appreciate both of you helping me out. I don't have anyone to turn to for help," she said wistfully. Looking at Sis, she said, "I think I've told you everything I know."

*She couldn't have had the wrong address. She had gone back outside three times to check the address of the building. There it was right over the front door, 420 Paca Street. Sharon had been up all night worrying about how Lily was doing. She had never been apart from Lily this long. Lily had to be there. She had to be OK. Sharon had knocked on the door gently at first, then harder and harder. She tried the doorknob when no one answered. The door opened easily and she immediately noticed the ominous quiet. The same dirty walls and filthy gray carpeting remained. A few chairs strewn haphazardly. Where only yesterday there had been a crowded waiting area, now quiet emptiness. Sharon felt she couldn't breathe. Stunned at first, she ran to the back of the room and through the door which led to the examining rooms.*

*Nothing. The horror of it hit her. Running now, fast, she checked each room. All four empty, no evidence that medical activities had taken place here. Frantic, she had run out of the room to check the address on the door, to look down the hall and then had run to check the outside of the building. Once on the street she looked up and down at the usual traffic of people and cars. The enormity of her loss consumed her. How would she ever find a tiny baby in all of humanity that was the city? How would she go on? Instinctively, she rushed back upstairs. Hoping she had been dreaming before, she again entered the apartment where she had last seen her baby. She walked into what had been the waiting room where she had spent her last hours with Lily and collapsed on the stained carpet hysterical.*

"I lay there for a long time," she said quietly. "Trying to figure out what to do. Then I went again into the examining room where I last held her." She paused, took a deep breath with a shudder and continued. "There was a trash can there. I threw up and then sat down on the floor—that ugly green and white linoleum floor and just closed my eyes and remembered how it was when Lily was in my arms. Her soft skin, her sweet smell like the freshest of air, her eyes that held such trust. I tried to imprint that in my mind. I know I went against the law by taking her there. I know I endangered her life. And now she is gone." Pleadingly she looked at Rufuos and then Sis, "What else could I have done? She was sick. And the doctors at the U.S. Government System Hospital said they couldn't do the surgery for at least two years. Two years!! The Underground said they could help her. I knew the government would not like what I had done, but I had no other choice."

"The Underground?" Rufuos said, "This doesn't sound like the Underground to me. This sounds like the Black Market."

"What do you mean? What's the difference?" her voice becoming more shrill. She felt her heart pounding in her throat.

"Well, the Black Market—they are just hoodlums with a little knowledge. They don't care what happens to you. Money, that's all that drives them, Ms. St. Clair. We have heard some pretty bad stuff regarding them." Rufuos said all of this apologetically.

"But I thought they were doctors. They should care."

"Well, there is an Underground," Rufuos cleared his throat and paused. But that's different."

"How do you mean?"

"Well, there is an organization that runs outside The U.S. Government Healthcare Distribution System but really does not function for profit. Altruistic you might say." Rufuos could no longer look at Sharon directly; he felt so guilty. He very well knew what had led Sharon to do what she had done. If he wasn't a police officer, he could easily have made the same mistake with Aaron.

"The Underground receives no press from any of the media sources," Rufuos continued. "All their websites are in code. You have to know them already, or have a connection, to get help from them." Rufuos stopped there, lowered and shook his head sadly.

Unfortunately, once again the higher levels of society found decent care, he thought to himself, while the Sharons of the world ended up with the very worst situations.

Rufuos hated being in situations where he had to lie or even keep anything hidden. Keeping Aaron's whereabouts secret from Sis was tough but necessary he felt—just like telling this woman that he might be able to help her find her baby was a huge stretch of the truth.

He looked up at Sis standing next to him and back at Sharon. "Do you have a fingerprint card for your baby?"

Sharon opened her purse and pulled out an envelope. "Here it is. Please find her. I'm begging you, please." She sat forward in her chair hopefully.

Rufuos had to give her that kernel of hope.

"Oh, and here," Sharon reached again into her purse and pulled out what looked like a round silver locket. "It's not real," she said sheepishly, "but look." She opened the round locket and revealed a picture of her baby. "Please take it."

Rufuos gently closed her tiny pale hand around the locket with his large brown, scarred hand. "Well, really, you can keep that. At this age, babies change awfully fast. The fingerprint is really all we need. We'll really try, Ms. St. Clair. We can't promise anything, but we'll really try. Maybe this organization simply relocated." That was as far as he could go. In his mind, Rufuos figured the baby would never be located. Lily would either turn up dead or had already been sold for adoption.

"Can I go?" Sharon looked from Sis to Rufuos unsure of what to do. "I mean, are you gonna arrest me for what I did?"

Rufuos looked at Sis who seemed about to say something, and said, "No, no, Ms. St. Clair. I don't think that will be necessary. Just stay home near your phone, so I can reach you. OK?"

"Oh!" she gasped. "Thank you. Thank you." She stood up to leave and looked at Sis. "Thank you also, Officer Leland. For listening to me." She reached for Sis' hand and, looking directly into Sis' eyes, shook it, "You have been so understanding. Thank you."

"Sure," Sis, eyes lowered, said quietly. And Sharon walked away.

"What was that about?" Sis asked Rufuos as soon as Sharon exited the squad room.

"What do you mean?" Rufuos looked up from the report Sis had already started earlier.

"I mean, since when do we just throw police procedure out with the wind?"

"What? You mean her? You wanted me to arrest her? Come on, Sis, she was desperate."

"I don't care. Do you realize what would happen if everyone did what she did? The whole U.S. Government Healthcare Distribution System would collapse. You just can't let people like that slide."

"Oh yeah? Really? People like that?" Rufuos put one hand on his hip and his jaw hardened. "I'm gonna at least try to find that baby," his voice deepened. "And I'm not gonna be judgmental."

Sis physically stepped back. In their five years on the job together Rufuos had never spoken to her like that.

He turned and headed for the door. He stopped and looked back at her, "Are you coming or not? Don't matter to me."

She sighed and quickly followed after.

# CHAPTER 23

Victor Swain saw nothing wrong in his Black Market connection. He viewed himself as a pragmatist. Any student of philosophy knew that morality was just a figment of man's imagination. God, an ancient myth, had for many years served as a controlling factor for society. But God was no more. And Victor believed he had been ahead of his time in his beliefs in self-fulfillment. He knew what people expected of him and he knew how to pretend. Ostensibly, he worked for the government to ensure a civilized approach to health services. But in reality he worked for himself. Expediency was the key. He used people as he believed they were meant to be used. Unfettered by questions of conscience, he freely and efficiently made decisions all day long, every day. And he only rose higher up the ladder of power. People in the lower rungs were simply incapable of making decisions. These lower level workers were necessary, of course, but truly expendable and inconsequential. He interacted with them only when he needed to. Like now. He needed to call Gail Tilden.

"A police officer? Are you sure he is a police officer's son?" Victor Swain sat up in his designer swivel armchair.

"Absolutely positive. The boy talks about his father all the time," Gail replied becoming more excited as Mr. Swain's interest increased. She looked out her window at St. Luke's steeple. "In fact, the father was here yesterday to see him. Wore his uniform and everything. Pretty bold, I'd say."

"Yes, certainly. Now Ms. Tilden I want you to keep this to yourself. Don't tell anyone else—no other agents, understood?"

"Yes, I understand completely. You can trust me totally. What do you want me to do?" And what other agents could he be referring to?

"Just keep an eye on the situation. I want to know if the boy is going to be discharged, in advance, if possible. The more advance time we have, the better. This is extremely helpful, Ms. Tilden. You might be in for an award for this." Might as well throw her a bone.

"Oh! Well, thank you, Mr. Swain. I'll certainly alert you to any changes here, and I'll keep a close eye on the boy, Aaron."

Victor hung up the phone and dialed another number connecting him once again inside St. Luke's. He was just finishing this latest conversation as Todd entered his office and sat down.

Victor looked up briefly to acknowledge Todd's arrival, "Her husband has just arrived. I will apprise him of his wife's progress. Glad you're there to keep an eye on things. I am getting updates from Gail as well. Don't worry. I will get you out before the government moves in for demolition."

At which Todd jumped up from his chair yelling "What? What about my wife."

"I'll talk to you later." Victor hung up the phone and looked placatingly at Todd. "Don't worry. I know you are concerned."

"Concerned! I'm way past concerned. When is my wife coming out of there? It's been four weeks. Now your government friends are going to be sending military people in there. I want her out. Just tell me where she is and I'll go get her."

"Calm down, Todd. No need for this. The government won't move until I tell them to. My mole at St. Luke's believes your wife will do well long-term from the treatment they are giving her. Stop worrying. I know you miss her. She'll be coming home soon from the sound of it. I don't know why you came over here anyway. It would be better if you didn't, you know."

"I came because of an email I received from my wife. I thought you should see it." With that Todd handed the paper over to Victor.


Dear Todd,

I miss you more than I can ever express with words. You are in my thoughts constantly. Please know that I am being treated medically in a way that I didn't know was possible. To have caring people listen to my complaints and explain each phase of my treatment is new to me. I wonder if these methods could not be used in the government hospitals? Of particular concern lately to me is realizing that all those who work here have the belief that the government is going to in some way destroy this facility. It is a diverse array of personalities running this place—not the least strange is the minister here who holds services each week for a small group of people.

Where they come from I don't know. The people here in the hospital have been kind to me even knowing that I represent the very organization that they believe wants to take their hospital away from them. I have told them that this is not true, but they refuse to accept what I say to them.

I'm hoping that you could help in this regard. Perhaps you could obtain a letter from Victor stating that the government has no plan to dismantle this organization. I understand they need to modify a bit what they are doing, but why wouldn't the government be willing to work with them to achieve parity with the City Wellness Centers? I am hopeful that you will be willing to assist with this.

I have missed you terribly. Hope you are well and look forward to coming home soon with good health.

Love,
Debra

"So, Victor, what do you think?"

"Look, Todd, she hasn't been well. She'll get over this. How can she really think clearly in her current state?"

"Maybe I should go see her?"

"NO! Absolutely not. We've got enough government people there as it is. We're working on getting them out. We don't need an ACLU lawyer in there mixing it up. Let's wait until she comes home. Then leave it to me. I will take care of St. Luke's. Nice and tidy without litigious lawyers like yourself."

"OK. I'll give you a little more time. But I want frequent updates concerning Deb's condition and an extraction date for her."

"I'll keep you informed." With that, Victor gave a dismissive nod toward the door indicating that the meeting was over. Todd took his cue reluctantly, and left.

Poor Todd, he seemed to be barely hanging on. Meanwhile things were falling into place for Victor Swain. He couldn't help feeling very satisfied with himself. Few people had the talent he had for juggling two very strong interest groups. Neither group had any idea, of course. He had control and in order to keep it, he needed his pawns to be clueless. Handling the government—he could do that in his sleep. The Black Market. That proved difficult all of the time and dangerous too much of the time lately. He needed to keep them in their place, to make them understand that they needed him and the government information he could provide. He knew both the Black Market and the U.S. Government wanted St. Luke's or at least, the supplies and equipment before the government came in.

If the trash hadn't piled up, the harbor might have even been scenic on a beautiful day like today. Waller didn't notice the mess around him; he made money whenever he came down to the harbor. Usually he didn't have to work that hard either. Today's client was an exception.

"I don't have any more," Waller said loudly. He wiped the juice that rolled down his chin, a result of saliva and the last piece of a hot dog. This guy just wouldn't quit. "Nothing more. I gave you more than you usually get."

"You're sure it's not going to the Underground—that Marcie chick?" Upon seeing the surprised look on Waller's face, "You think we don't know? Don't insult me and my organization, Waller. We know everything about you. We know you are incapable of loyalty. But we will continue paying you well, very well. Stay with us and get rich, or desert us and, well, it won't be good for you, not good for you at all."

"Now who could he be? Do you recognize him, Sis?" Rufuos had calmed down considerably. They were sitting in a coffee shop located on the water at Baltimore Harbor. They had come looking for Waller and had not been disappointed. They planned to question him and had even started out of the coffee shop to do just that, coffee in hand, when the other fellow had arrived. And a strange one he was too. Tall, much taller than Waller, who must have been getting a crick in his neck looking up at the stranger. The stranger had slicked back his black hair so that his head shone in the sunlight. He kept his hands in the pockets of his three quarter length black leather look jacket. Did he have his hand on a gun? Rufuos naturally wondered.

"He's turning!" Sis said excitedly. Together they groaned when as he turned, the fact that he had on mirrored sunglasses became apparent.

"I hate those!" Rufuos said vehemently. The face turned in their direction and stared. Weirdly, the two officers stared back and finally looked down at their coffee as they both realized connecting in such a way with this man could prove unhealthy.

The man turned again and sauntered away. Sis and Rufuos looked up and watched him until he disappeared up Calvert Street beyond their view. Rufuos quickly looked back to where the discussion had taken place and, noticing Waller gone, sprang to action.

"Come on, Sis. We've got to talk to the Waller guy."

"Right behind you," she replied panting as she ran after Rufuos. The officers arrived together at the spot where they had seen Waller and looked frantically in all directions. Simultaneously, they spotted Waller.

Back at the hot dog stand.

"Of course," Sis whispered, "Let's grab him!" They walked quietly up to Waller who was busy spreading mustard on his two hot dogs. Sis grabbed an arm while Rufuos put his face nose to nose with Waller.

"Hey, you almost made me drop this!" a surprised and indignant Waller cried.

Rufuos said, "We need some advice."

"Aw, come on, I don't know anything that can help you. I'm small potatoes." Waller continued preparing his hot dogs.

"Okay, you know nothing," Sis moved in closer. "What nothing were you discussing with the man who just left?" Waller squirmed, his eyes darting back and forth between the two.

Sis took another step toward him, "Yeah, we know. Nothing is nothing. But pain is something. What did he want and who is he?"

"Look, I'm trying to stay in business here." Waller used his best wheedling voice. "You wouldn't want me going on welfare, would you?"

"A name, Waller," Rufuos said calmly.

"Just a name," Sis narrowed her eyes, and hissed.

"If you think we have to let you go, you're wrong. We can keep you," Rufuos added.

"In fact, we want to," Sis interrupted.

"We think you're cute," Rufuos added sweetly.

"Oh sure, oh sure," Waller babbled nervously.

"Just a name is all we want. We could stop the man himself and ask him," Sis said.

"Well, why don't you?" Waller asked haughtily and proceeded to take a huge bite of his hot dog.

"Oh, because you're here, and we're such good friends," Sis looped her arm around Waller's as if they were the best of buddies. "We don't want you to feel left out. We like to keep our friends close, know what I mean?" She tightened her grip on Waller.

"Well, I don't want to be included, thank you very much." Waller replied. "I don't want any friends neither. So, go away." He tried to slip out of Sis' grasp, but she used both arms to hang on and gave a little yank.

At Waller's surprised gasp, Sis said simply, "Weight training." She smiled cynically, "Oh, we will be going. We will just want to see if maybe a visit to a new friend might be in order. Make sure you're not getting him into trouble."

"Me? Me getting him into trouble? I don't think so. This guy will hurt me bad if he finds out I talked to you. He's probably watching us right now." Waller looked around nervously. "Now, you gotta protect me."

"Of course we will." Now soothing, Sis spoke gently into his ear. "You will be safe. Don't worry. So, who is he?"

He tried, "Wouldn't you like to know?" but seeing Sis' eyes narrow and feeling the pain in his arm increase, he gave in, "That, that is the head of the Black Market Medicine Organization." Waller smiled triumphantly.

"Well, that's very interesting. He must have a lot of interest in you if he came to see you in person."

"Oh yeah, a lot. He wanted drugs. That's all he ever wants. Whatever he wants, I try to give it to him. I try to keep him happy. I have to. Much as I can 'cause I know he means business." Waller kept his eyes on his rapidly disappearing hot dog.

"Waller, I can't believe you are dealing with those guys." Rufuos used his I'm your best friend voice. "I have heard some serious stuff about the Black Market group. Former techies aren't they? Mixed in with plenty of drug use. Have some issues. Besides their desire to make money, don't they have a personality problem? You know, they like to kill people. Have you met with him before?"

"Oh, plenty of times," Waller bragged. "He comes to me for advice. He respects me." He stuffed the rest of the hot dog in his sloppy mouth.

"Oh, right. Respect. And I'll just bet you respect him."

Waller nodded chewing noisily. "Now you got it."

"Waller, you're lucky to be alive," Rufuos said disgustedly. "Lucky to be alive. Did he mention a baby?"

"A baby?" Waller, paused, looked up off into the distance and then back at Rufuos, "No, not at all."

"This particular baby was a patient of one of his quack doctors. The mother dropped her off at a clinic and the next day returning for her baby discovers—no baby and no clinic or any sign of life at the clinic. What do you know of this, Waller?"

"Nothing! I know absolutely nothing about no baby. Besides that's small potatoes. I told you, Cyrus Kadar only deals in big things." Sis and Rufuos glanced at each other. Rufuos plowed on before Waller could think of what he was saying.

"Well, it isn't nothing to the mother of that baby. If not the baby, what did you talk about?"

"Oh, nothing much."

"Yeah, we know, that nothing word again," Sis said disgustedly.

Rufuos grabbed a napkin out of Waller's hand and roughly wiped the mustard colored juice out of the corner of Waller's mouth. "You better come clean with this one. A lot of lives depend on you. Lives that are a lot more valuable than your own, Waller." Rufuos paused. "That's just the nature of things. You understand." Rufuos stuffed the soiled napkin into Waller's shirt pocket.

"Yeah, yeah I get your drift. OK, you have to keep this to yourselves. Do we have an agreement on that?"

"Yeah, you have our word as police officers. It will all be kept a secret."

"Even from the other cops. I mean this guy would hurt me bad if this got out."

"OK, you got a deal. Now what did this Cyrus Kadar guy want."

"Well, of course, like I said, he's looking for drugs. They always are. They pay well, so usually it's no problem, but I've been having a little problem lately finding the ones they want. It's not so easy what I do. Maybe some day you'll realize that and treat me with a little more respect."

"That's all? That's all you've got?"

"What?"

"What?! You haven't given us anything. I feel like hauling you into a holding cell just for fun, Waller." Rufuos glanced to Sis for agreement.

"You know he's not worth it. He'll just stink up our car," Sis said nonchalantly.

"What? I told you all I know," Waller looked as if Sis had let her best friend down.

"Yeah, well, so much for you being on the inside track, Waller. 'Cause you know what? You know nothing. Nada. Zip. You've been no help. A fact which my partner and I will not forget. Got it, mister? Nothing." Rufuos gave Waller a quick shove. "Come on, Sis. Let's get away from this thing." And the two walked away from a very relieved Waller.

"Okay, so at least we got a name." Heading back to their car Sis couldn't keep from giggling. "He is such a jerk and stupid."

"Yeah, he still doesn't realize he gave us a name. Where could this Cyrus Kadar guy go after getting the bad news from Waller? If Waller was telling the truth, he has given the guy no medicine for the Black Market. That would mean that Cyrus Kadar would need to continue on to find some medicine. Because his organization needs medical supplies and equipment to survive. Computers aren't a problem since the techies have plenty of those. But special medicines and testing tools such as an MRI are harder to find."

"He has to have the medicines. We know that," Sis said. "A lot of the other stuff they can do without, but when it comes to the medicines, well, they just have to have that or they are out of business. So who do we know besides Waller who deals with medicine?"

"Marcie, how about her?" Rufuos said hesitantly.

"She could be helpful, but we don't have an address on her."

"Yeah. That's OK. We'll try to guess where she will go," Rufuos said as he started the engine of the police cruiser.

"I know where her first stop usually is," Sis said with a smile, "Salmund's office, right? I think she may be a little sweet on him."

"You're kidding, right? They seem different as night and day to me. Besides, you're on shift and the private lives of people like Marcie are none of our concern."

"Oh, sure, but I think it would be nice if they got together," Sis leaned her head back and closed her eyes. "After I arrest them and put them in jail, of course."

"Naturally," Rufuos replied as he turned up Calvert Street to head for Matthew Salmund's office.

# CHAPTER 24

Marcie's intense eyes missed nothing about Matthew's office. From his diplomas behind his desk to the window overlooking the squash courts. His desk, always immaculate, took up one entire wall of the spacious office. The desk, metallic silver, buffed to such a shine that Marcie could gaze appraisingly into her hazel colored beady eyes. She had always wished that her eyes were larger, but today they seemed to hold her whole reflection.

Marcie didn't often peer inside herself, but events of late made her feel she needed more in her life. She had never kidded herself about her unimportance in the world. On the contrary, she prided herself in her ability to survive and remain self-reliant. She had no special mission in life. Not like Matthew, who determined early in his life to make a positive contribution to society. Marcie had no such altruistic motivation. Or so she had thought. Until now. For years, her life had revolved around the routine of procurement. But now looking at her reflection as she waited for Matthew to finish his report, she realized that her activity provided more than just money. More, even, than self-importance. People relied on her. Her job meant something, actually quite a lot, to some. Until now, she had thought Matthew somewhat a minimal man, too concerned with righteous anger. Startled, she saw now that they were much the same. Maybe not outwardly, but inside. She studied him. His head bent, Matthew put the finishing touches on some paperwork and then looked up. His eyes held defeat.

"I really don't want to close St. Luke's."

"I know," Marcie said softly.

"I just don't see how we can save it. We've got at least two government agents out there. Not to mention a senator."

"I know. It's a little crowded with high profile people. But don't you think maybe the senator could help?"

"Well, obviously she could if she wanted to. But if she is like the others, she just wants her needs met, and then out she will go, never looking back."

"It's disappointing. I thought she might be different," Marcie said quietly.

Suddenly attentive, Matthew said, "Are you going soft, Marcie?" Marcie's eyes flickered in embarrassment. She hesitated, then looked at Matthew directly.

"Maybe I am," then looking away, "I wonder if I could persuade her."

Matthew sat back in his chair and taking a breath said, "You want to take a stab at it? You're a woman. She's a woman. Maybe you can do what Reverend McClaren could not. We have some time. As long as they keep her there, the government won't come in."

The door abruptly swung open with Melody's loud "You can't go in there" voice following the two officers. Sis and Rufuos strode purposefully into the room each coming to a stop on either side of Matthew's desk.

"So, Marcie and Matthew! Rufuos gave them each a cheery smile. What a team! Are you expanding your horizons?"

"How dare you barge in here without my say so! You've just broken procedure set by your own organization." Matthew spoke with authority and calm, but Marcie noticed the tension in his face.

Sis said, "Yeah, we do that sometimes."

Matthew stood indicating with a raised hand in her direction to Marcie to stay put and be silent.

"When we suspect Black Market activity, we can barge in wherever we deem necessary," Sis continued.

"We have nothing to do with any type of Black Market activities," Matthew said slowly and distinctly.

"There's that word again," Rufuos said shaking his head. But he made no eye contact with either Matt or Marcie.

"Yeah," Sis said, not taking her eyes off Matthew. "Yeah 'nothing' just keeps popping up."

Matthew sat back down. "I know of no such place as this, what do you call it, St. Luke's."

"Oh, really?" Sis put a hand on her hip. "We have followed you there. Both of you actually. It didn't seem unfamiliar to you at that time."

Marcie looked up at this point for the first time noticing Rufuos. Her intense round eyes grew. What was going on here? He wouldn't look in her direction. In fact he wasn't looking anywhere except at his partner.

Matthew glanced at Rufuos who was hanging back and letting Sis lead the charge. He looked only at Sis when he said, "OK, so we know about St. Luke's, but you've got it wrong. It's not a part of the Black Market. It's the Underground. It has nothing to do with the Black Market. All services are free. You can't have a black market when nothing is for sale. All services are volunteered; all moneys are charitably given. You have no evidence we are connected with anybody else. You couldn't possibly because we aren't."

"Why don't you try Waller?" Marcie said suddenly.

"Funny you should mention him," Sis responded. "Already been there. He had little to say. Nothing really." Sis said thoughtfully. She had noticed Rufuos' lack of participation. What was with him? First, he wanted to get at these guys, and now he was holding back.

She managed to restrain her anger until Rufuos took his coat off and slung it over the chair at his desk back at the station.

"OK, what's going on Rufe? I have a right to know. I am your partner, you know. What gives with you? You're running hot and cold on this, and that makes me very uneasy, especially since it just isn't like you to be this way. Do you want to get this Underground or not?"

"Well, it's just not so simple," Rufuos sat down with a sigh.

"Yeah, when did it become not simple? Tell me! Let me in on what is going on in that mind of yours."

"Can't you just trust me on this one, Sis? It's better for you if you don't know what's going on."

"OK, that's it. Something is going on, isn't it? Well, I damn sight better be told and right now." She sat down opposite him where the perp usually sat and said, "OK I'm listening."

Rufuos looked at her and then said, "Just let me think a minute."

"No!" she yelled and heads turned. She looked around the room and lowered her voice. "No thinking! Just talk or I'll take you into the captain right now. You're tensing up, and that makes me tense, and when cops get nervous, they make mistakes. You know that, Rufe. You know you have got to come clean with me. And now, while we're not in the thick of it."

"OK. OK. But not here. Too many people watching. Let's go for a drive. OK?"

The computer hummed softly alive but with no eyes to the world, only inward.

New mail: This place is crawling with unknowns. The environment continues to be unstable. Are you keeping me totally informed? No more surprises.

Reply: Be advised I sent no one to visit. Must be coincidence.

Reply: I don't have these kinds of friends. Just be sure to call off your troops until I have a chance to sort things out. I don't like this sort of activity.

Paul's computer had served its usefulness time and again with the surveillance email program he had installed. Who was that? Paul checked the email address followed the links to … St. Luke's! They did have someone in there. And it wasn't Gail. He knew all about her, including her email addresses. Paul had been dozing in front of the computer when he tapped into an email conversation between someone at St. Luke's and Swain. Sounded like communication between the two wasn't too good. This was news, not for the internet but definitely news. Paul copied the emails and then immediately began burying the transmission that he had worked so hard to find.

While he cleaned up the previous transmission, the screen began speaking again.

This time Paul knew who all the parties were:

New mail: It's time to get her out. (Hartman)

Reply: Don't worry. I am keeping informed. (Swain)

New mail: The Black Market wants in and you are dragging your feet. (Kadar)

Reply: You will hear from me soon enough. (Swain)

New mail: I don't want her anywhere near there when things break. (Hartman)

Reply: I have this under control. (Swain)

Paul whistled to himself as he saved this exchange and then deleted the information from the hard drive.

That done he grabbed his backup clip and his jacket and headed out the door. McClaren needed to know who he was dealing with. Things hadn't seemed so difficult when it was just the government they were worried about. It was time to move. St. Luke's was in trouble, and Paul had to make McClaren and the others see that. Paul paused, returned to his computer and sent a message to Matt, "Meet me out there. You know where I mean. ASAP. I'm going now."

Breaking into a run as soon as he got out of his news office, Paul jumped into his car and headed to outcountry. Was he being followed? He didn't know, but didn't think it mattered anyway. When information made it to the government, you couldn't hide anywhere. They would have to deal. And Matthew was the man for that. He had done it before. Paul knew where his own shortcomings were. He was a computer nerd. Matt knew how to negotiate. It would take Matt's best skills to handle the Black Market and The U.S. Government. Matt always said it was no big deal. Just figure out what everybody wanted, and then try to find a way for everyone to get what they wanted or at least think they did. So as near as Paul could tell, the Black Market wanted drugs and equipment for their operation. McClaren and his gang of idealists wanted a place to conduct their hospital in peace. The government mainly wanted everything kept quiet.

In the short term, of course. They wanted St. Luke's dismantled because the senator had been there. But in the long term it seemed fine with government if these outcountry hospitals (the Underground) kept popping up. Everyone, including members of Congress, liked to think there was a good place to go when you were really sick even if it was illegal to do so. The Black Market was losing credibility fast. It had initially maintained a superior standard of care. But that was no more. Money was the only thing for them now. The government didn't care that they existed. Why?

Paul had his own theory as to why the government allowed the Black Market to exist. The Black Market could do the dirty work like dozing St. Luke's. Nobody in the city was going to know or care about St. Luke's, but if they did investigate, it would be the Black Market that the violent destruction would be linked back to and not the government.

Meanwhile, if a government official needed meds or treatment, the Black Market could always find it for them and supply whatever was needed should the chosen outcountry clinic be short of supplies. Which they always were. He knew that from what Matt had told him.

So if it's drugs they want, that's what they would have to give them. The Black Market could be satisfied. After all, it was to their benefit for the current method of drug procurement to stay functional.

# Chapter 25

Once a place died, hopelessness set in in the apparent form of its residents. Baltimore harbor, once a place bustling with activity and culture, had died long ago. For every three boarded up businesses, there remained one half-way house or struggling business. The people struggled too. Shabbily dressed, they wandered aimlessly, their vacant eyes looking off on the horizon perhaps thinking relief could be found there. It couldn't. Broken down, peeling benches provided their only comfort. No one cared that a once thriving metropolis had deteriorated into a city desert. Barren of life and activity, it served only as a home to the lonely and lost. People unable to see a way to success came here. At least they found others like themselves. They didn't have to look at others who had succeeded. Who wanted to be reminded of failure? The police didn't even bother you down here. There really was no one to rob. No one had anything.

Sis and Rufuos headed for the harbor whenever they had something to discuss. Only here could they be uninterrupted. Here no one cared what they were saying.

"So, OK. We're in the car." Sis looked out over the harbor. Nothing but bums around. "So what's the scoop, Rufe. What are you hiding from me?"

"I know you're not going to like this. But just listen. Hear me out before you get excited."

"OK. OK. Tell me already!"

"You know Aaron?"

"Yes, your son?"

"Yeah, Aaron, my son. Haven't you wondered why we haven't invited you over lately?"

"Well, yeah, kind of, I just figured you were busy."

"Yes, that's true. We've been busy. Stacey and I and the kids too. But that isn't the reason. The real reason is if you had come over, you would have seen that Aaron wasn't there."

Alarmed, Sis sat up. "Is he OK?"

"Yeah, *now* he is OK." Rufuos paused. "No thanks to the U.S. Government Healthcare System. They told me I could have nothing because of the time when the others were sick. Remember that? And then Stacey had to have her operation. They told me we would have to wait. So I thought OK. He's young and strong; he can wait. But when I put his diagnosis through a hospital computer program, I got back info that said we shouldn't wait. So I tried again. Sis, I really tried to do it legal. But no way. They didn't care about his age or what might happen if we waited. Even that it would be more expensive if we waited. To tell you the truth, I don't think they ever intended to help us. Ever. Sis, do you know what that means?"

"I think I do, and I have a feeling where you're headed."

"I had to try something else. Remember that young mother? I know just how she felt. Why she would have done what she did. I probably would have done the same, but I'm a whole lot luckier than that poor girl 'cause I knew about the Underground. I even had someone to lead me there."

"Marcie."

"Yep! Marcie. That's right—took me right to St. Luke's. Remember how I missed some days? I followed her right to St. Luke's. And they took my Aaron in. And he is getting better. I would be willing to go to jail for him. I really would, but is it right for me to go to jail? Have I really done anything wrong?" He sighed heavily and said, "I'm just asking you to think about it."

"It doesn't matter if you think it's right. You know that, Rufe. It matters that what you did is illegal. You're a police officer. Others don't get to do what you're doing. This is wrong."

"Try to understand. I know it's hard." Rufuos lowered his voice. "You don't have kids and all. But when it's your kid, you'll do anything."

"That's why the laws are tough. It's inconsiderate—you taking the healthcare when someone else might need it and be entitled to it."

"You know all that sounds just dandy when you are not responsible for someone else's care. I'm the only help that boy has, and I will search to the ends of the earth and pay whatever I got to pay to help him. He's my kid."

Sis put her head in her hands. "What am I going to do?"

"I don't know. What are you going to do?"

"How can we continue to work together if I know you'll go outside the law?"

"Aw, Sis, come on. You know I'm a good man. I know the difference between right and wrong."

"Do you? Really? I'm not so sure you do, Rufe. Where else will you fudge the law? I think you better take me back to the station house. I'm putting in for a new partner. Today."

They were silent on the ride back. Rufe dropped Sis at the door as was his custom. As she got out, he said, "What are you going to tell them? What reason are you going to give them?"

"I don't know yet. What difference does it make to you?" And she slammed the car door and walked off not looking back even though Rufe thought she would.

Rufe pulled the squad car into the garage. He got out of the car and headed for his locker in the station house. He knew what the rules said. Sis would have to write him up.

He stopped before entering the building and made a quick decision. He dialed his wife on his cell phone. "Stacey, we gotta move. Remember how I told you we might? Well, we gotta now. So follow the plan like we discussed and meet me where I told you. Yeah, just go pick up the kids. And meet me like we said. We're going to be all right, just remember that. We'll be OK."

Downstairs at St. Luke's the hospital was a bustle of activity. "Just in case" preparations were being made to go at a moment's notice. Senator Debra Jamison watched in amazement from the doorway of her room as the various teams of doctors and nurses checked each patient, put supplies with each patient rather than having them locked up in a central location as usual. It was eerily quiet as everyone worked. In their effort to keep the patients calm, the doctors and nurses had inadvertently created a silent environment of fear. St. Luke's was usually a lot noisier with conversations and directions going on.

Upstairs, McClaren prayed in the darkened sanctuary. His eyes closed. His hand over his brow. As if he could shut out the world. The answer came from the book of Ephesians, 1:18, "The eyes of your understanding being enlightened; that ye may know what is the hope of his calling … " Then he arose and headed to his office for the meeting Paul had called to decide the fate of St. Luke's and the medical staff and patients within.

Chambers was already there with John standing by his side. Marilyn walked in with Matthew and Marcie who had just arrived. McClaren took his place at his desk. Suddenly there was a doorbell. Marilyn said, "I'll go."

"Now who could that be? They can't be here already," John said.

"We still have the senator. Don't think they'll bother you 'til she goes home," Chambers said pointedly. "I haven't released her yet. She's been asking but I keep putting her off. I don't like it, but that's what I've been doing ... " his voice trailed off and he looked down at the floor.

"And we know you feel compromised. We appreciate it, as do all the patients here and the staff do as well." McClaren said kindly. "Paul will be here soon. Ah, here is Marilyn." He smiled warmly at her as she entered.

"You have some guests," Marilyn said as she entered the room. She saw McClaren's worried look. "I told them to sit in the sanctuary."

"OK, don't keep us in suspense. Who is it?" Marcie asked.

"Aaron's mother and two sisters have arrived to visit him. I told them we were in a meeting. She said she would be fine waiting there. Didn't think you wanted them downstairs just yet. Her husband being a police officer and all."

"Good, that will be fine," McClaren said relieved. "Where shall we begin? Ah, good, here comes Paul. Just the person I wanted to start with."

Paul stepped into the now crowded little room and looked around at those in attendance. "Hello, Reverend. Sorry I'm a bit late. I wanted to hide my tracks—on my computer that is."

"OK," McClaren smiled, "Well, we're all here to decide what should be our next course of action. Paul says he has some new information."

"Yes," Paul went on to describe the connection between Swain and Hartman.

"Does the senator know?" John asked. "She seems too nice to be a part of all that."

"I can't answer that question just now. Don't know where she stands. And we do have to be careful." Paul hesitated. "Actually there is a leak from within our organization." Everyone looked around the room uncomfortably and a number of eyes rested on John.

"What? It isn't me," he said indignantly. "I'm just married to her. I never worked as a spy for the government."

Paul immediately jumped in with, "The government contact I'm concerned about is not Ms. Tilden. Though I suspect she would like to think she was." Paul gave a wry smile to everyone after glancing pointedly at John. "So, what shall we do?"


"See you tomorrow Sis," Rufuos said as he slammed his locker shut and placed his cap on his head, eyes averted.

"Yep! See you tomorrow." Sis wouldn't look up. They both knew she wasn't leaving yet. She had a report to write.

She can't help it, Rufe told himself as he hurried to his car. Hopefully, Stacey had followed his instructions, and they would all be together soon. He would miss the department and his job, and, yes, even Sis who at this moment was writing him up for not carrying out his duties aggressively and with integrity. He didn't care. Sis couldn't possibly understand his predicament. Oh, sure, she acted as if she understood like when she was talking with Ms. St. Clair. But she really didn't know what the feeling was. That feeling of total impotence. The total lack of power when someone trusted you and you let him down and that someone was your son. Well, he wasn't going to let Aaron down or Stacey or his daughters for that matter. They came before a bunch of departmental regulations. His wheels spun out as he took the curve out of the parking lot and headed out of the station parking lot.

"Mommy, is Aaron here? Are we going to get to see him?" Donna, seven years old, with dark curls and huge eyes tugged impatiently on the sleeve of her mother's blue corduroy jacket. "It's spooky in here. Do we have to stay? Couldn't we just wait in the car?"

"No!" her mother answered impatiently, "Daddy told us definitely to come inside. We have to do what Daddy wanted us to do." Then, catching herself, Stacey said more kindly, "Now hush up. Give me a chance to think. This is kind of a strange place. Here, hold me close, Donna. And take Karyn's hand." Donna took her four year old sister's hand—the one she wasn't sucking on and looked back up at her mother who said, "That's it. We'll all stay together and wait for Daddy. He'll be here. I just don't know when. Try to be patient."

"And so will I," Stacey thought to herself. "Please, get here Rufuos. I don't know these people, and I want to see Aaron."

# CHAPTER 26

Gail had always believed in the order of the universe. Beyond that, she figured no one knew. Her sense of order pervaded her observations of people and how she did her job. Indeed, she saw herself as someone who helped to maintain order so that life could be reasonably good (i.e. ordered) for everyone. Gail defined crime as disorder. In her job she tried to replace disorder with order and calm. Civilization depended on regulation. Who could possibly argue with that? She had already admitted to herself that St. Luke's operated in a far more orderly fashion than she ever suspected. Unfortunately, they took an ordered medical plan and placed it in a disordered region. This couldn't be right. She knew she couldn't convince anyone here at St. Luke's of this. They all could be working for the government, and doing far more good than they were doing out here in the middle of nowhere. She sighed and sat down at her desk.

Finally, Gail could use the computer without interruption. Everyone seemed to be in McClaren's office right now, except for the patients, of course. Using the computer she dialed Mr. Swain's number. The phone rang only twice before Mr. Swain, her contact, picked up.

"There seems to be a change coming," she said over the phone after exchanging niceties with Mr. Swain.

"You've done a fine job, Ms. Tilden. We know they are up to something."

"Did you know Senator Jamison is here?"

"No, I didn't," Swain faked sincere surprise and interest.

"She's been here for quite some time actually, I only recently found out about it," Gail lied.

"Really? What's she there for?"

"Some strange illness. I don't know why she came here when she could have stayed right near home and used a government facility," Gail said somewhat irritably.

"Who can explain the rich and powerful, Ms. Tilden? Certainly not you and not I. We are merely government servants. But you know all this already."

"Yes, I do know what you mean," Gail said respectfully. "Well, there is certainly a lot of preparation going on here for something. I'm sorry to say that I don't know what."

"Don't worry, Ms. Tilden. You are doing a great job there. The government is extremely grateful to you, Ms. Tilden."

Gail paused. Swain's behavior bothered her. His comments did not reflect his usual demanding way. "What else could I do for you?" she asked frowning.

"Well, since you asked. I would like you to check into something else. I'm going to email you a list of medicines and ask you to see if you can take a look around, discreetly, of course, and let me know the quantities and locations of these medicines. The government would certainly be happy to have this information."

Gail paused for a moment and looked questioningly at the receiver before she said, "I'll be happy to do it, sir, but I wonder how much longer everything is going to be here. I think they are thinking of making a move as I have already reported."

"You let me worry about that Ms. Tilden. I'm sure the government has reasons for wanting this information. Be sure you delete and bury the email once you have memorized the medicines." Swain added the memorization comment on a silly whim. This lady was so dumb. She would do anything for a promotion. Anything except think, which made his job a whole lot easier. "I think we've talked on signal long enough, Ms. Tilden, don't you?"

"Oh, yes sir. I'll send the information on the encrypted wireless when I have it."

"Very good. And Ms. Tilden, let's keep this just between the two of us and, again, thank you from the United States Government."

Ms. Tilden plopped down on her bed with an unattractive scowl on her face and gazed intensely at her computer. Since when did her job entail spying and keeping information from other government agencies? Gail found herself suspecting Swain—of what she didn't know at this point. But if the government wanted medicine and supplies from St. Luke's, why didn't they just come and take them. And there was something else. Up until today, Gail had had the distinct impression that Swain couldn't stand her, but today he had been buttering her up for this drug thing. What would he do with the information once she compiled the list of medicines? Where were they going? He obviously planned to use the medicines for something. And he didn't plan to use customary channels. Disorder. She hated it.

# CHAPTER 27

Once a place of routine, the hospital's activities were becoming more and more unpredictable. Senator Jamison had grown used to the rhythm of the average day at St. Luke's. The doctors and nurses all came around at the same time of day with the same questions. Her health showed major improvement. Each day she grew stronger and thus less afraid to track her health by her appearance in the mirror that she kept in the toiletry case next to her bed. She reached for her little round mirror now and took a good look. The age lines were still there but her eyes, they were definitely brighter now. Was the disease receding, or was it finally having hope that made her eyes seem alive?

"So, what do you think?" She looked past the mirror to see John Macklin standing at the foot of her bed.

"I am pleased."

"Your labwork came back." He had the printouts in his hand.

"And?"

He smiled and came over to her, handed her the papers. "Dr. Chambers can explain all this better than I can. But it looks very good." And Senator Jamison looked good. "How do you feel?"

"Better than I have in a very long time. I feel like I could jump out of this bed and do all sorts of things. My energy has been so low up until now."

"Yep, you are definitely improving. No question about that."

"Thank you, John."

"Oh, don't thank me. Thank Dr. Chambers."

"I certainly shall."

"I've got some other stuff to do. I'll check in a little later."

Senator Jamison held out her hand, and John reached forward to hold it.

"Thank you," she whispered.

John just nodded and patted the top of her hand. Then he left to continue his rounds.

Debra closed her eyes, not to sleep, but just to relax and savor the moment.

"I hope I'm not intruding." A hesitant voice came from the edge of her bed. Jamison opened her eyes and saw a young lady.

"Of course not. I always welcome visitors," she answered warmly. "There are precious few out here."

"We haven't met."

"Ah yes, I know, but this being the small place that it is, I know who you are, Ms. Tilden."

"I really came here just to find my husband."

"Really? You just missed him. He was here just a few minutes ago," Senator Jamison stared, her eyebrows raised in a question.

"OK, so maybe I wanted to find him, and maybe I didn't. Maybe, I just wanted to shake things up a bit."

"And have you?"

"Maybe. But maybe I'm the one feeling unsteady."

"So, you came to see me. To see if I am feeling unsteady. Interesting. Have you learned anything while you have been here, Ms. Tilden?"

"Actually, yes, I have. And I confess I am confused."

"Join the club. Imagine how I feel. I didn't really want to come here in the first place. My husband insisted, said I owed it to my voters. But what a hypocrite I am. Totally. So are you going to have to turn me in? Should I be afraid of you, Ms. Tilden?"

"Actually, I don't really know. We are supposed to be on the same side. I'm supposed to be totally against what is happening here. It's just ... I don't know. It doesn't feel wrong to me. Before being here, I had a sense of what I was doing and why. Now, I don't know; it's very confusing. I'm used to a calm, uneventful life, not the unpredictable. And I never imagined that I would see the value in a place like this. The very type of place I'm trying to destroy. And now, Senator, I'm starting to wonder who I'm destroying it for."

"Really? What do you mean?"

"My boss, just now, I talked with him. His behavior is odd and noncommittal to say the least. I don't know what his goals are, where he's headed with all of this. I really need to not feel like a hypocrite, Senator Jamison. I need to know that my job is valuable. That it matters what I do. I know John doesn't think I care about right and wrong. But I do."

"Something big *is* troubling you?"

"Oh very big. My boss." Gail quietly pulled the makeshift curtain around the senator's bed and moved closer. Her voice was soft. "Here is the thing. Can I trust you? Really trust you not to reveal the information I am about to give you? Because this could be bad for me." She pulled her hand uncharacteristically through her hair. Her normally perfectly groomed hair now a mess, she continued, "You see I don't understand who I'm dealing with anymore. I used to understand the world. I used to understand what my life meant, what work meant. Even John, my husband, I thought I understood him. But now I don't know. I'm not sure about anything. It's like first one thing and then the next. What else don't I know I keep wondering." She stopped, looked directly at Debra and heaving a sigh said, "Do you understand anything I am saying, or is it all just gibberish?"

"Oh no, you are making a lot of sense to me," Debra responded thoughtfully. "I too am confused. After all, I helped create this health system, inadvertently, of course. I really believed in what I was doing. Now I'm wondering how many people have I hurt? And how unfair it is for me to be safe and sound here at St. Luke's when others die simply because they can't be treated, by law, a law which I helped create. My husband helped me rationalize it before I got here. If I become president, I could have a tremendous effect, but do the ends justify the means? I don't know. This is what I wonder about. They are getting ready to move. I know they fear the government. Yet look how good they have been to me. No one has chastised me for what I did. They all struggle as the government makes delivering care harder for them. But still they go ahead with what they are doing. Taking a huge risk. I too have my doubts and confusion that I didn't have before coming here. You could say that they are putting on a show for us. But I don't really believe that. So we are both confused; why don't you give me some information. What did your supervisor say to you that has disturbed you so?"

"He wants me to send him a list. A list of the supplies here. I ask myself why does he want that information? The government could come in here and take whatever they wanted. Why have me do it?"

"Why indeed?"

"What are you thinking?"

"Unfortunately, I'm thinking I do have a suspicion." The senator appeared deeply troubled. "Who is your contact?"

Gail told her.

A visibly shaken Jamison replied softly and more to herself than to Gail, "He is connecting with another organization. We'll talk later," she said suddenly with a dismissive attitude.

As soon as Gail left, Debra, energized, jumped out of bed and began getting dressed. Was Swain getting involved with the Black Market now? Or worse, was he dealing on his own? Was this an isolated case? Or had he been dirty all along? Jamison took a good look at her face as she visited the bathroom. She saw determination.

McClaren's crowded office was silent. Each person seemed absorbed in his or her own thoughts. McClaren looked from Dr. Chambers to Paul then to John and Marilyn. Even Marcie seemed to be staring at the floor lost in her own world. McClaren grew impatient.

"So what will we do?" he said to the group. Each looked to the other. Realizing that he would have to be the one to make the decision, McClaren said, "I've heard no other viable options. We will have to move."

Paul backed him up. "It really is time to make a move."

"I have found two other outcountry sites. We will have to split up since neither one has room for all of us. I believe the doctors should group the patients according to their needs and make the decision as to which patient goes to which place. Dr. Chambers, are you willing to supervise that effort?"

"Certainly," Chambers replied.

"I know you have been ready for this move, Dr. Chambers. Actually you can leave at this point. John will go with you and help with the organization for your task." John looked up, happy to be given a role in the move.

"Perhaps I should help." Marilyn offered watching the two leave.

"Oh, no! I don't think that would be wise," Paul said.

McClaren felt disappointment tug inside his chest. Paul's behavior meant only one thing. His eyes connected with Paul's, and he knew he was right. Paul had wisely moved to block the doorway. Marilyn looked over at Marcie and Matt. Marcie's dark eyes glared back at her, and Matt's expression held pure contempt.

Only Paul remained outwardly unemotional. "How much time do we have?" he asked quietly.

"They will come for the senator tomorrow," Marilyn answered.

"The senator won't be here," Debra Jamison said assuredly from the doorway.


"You know that wasn't part of the deal," Swain said struggling to keep calm. He had met Cyrus Kadar for lunch at their usual meeting place.

"Things change, Swain. You know that. Surely you didn't expect my organization to sit by and watch the government destroy a site that could be a lucrative business. One which we could handle very well. There are plenty of medical personnel in our organization who would be happy to have one of our own hospitals to work in."

"You're asking for trouble here, Cyrus." Swain tried a reasonable tact. "The government is not going to allow this. You have got to know that."

Cyrus Kadar, who had been intently interested in his steak sandwich, swallowed, took a sip of water and looked directly into Swain's eyes. "The government may be able to keep a lid on the Underground, but they cannot possibly control the Black Market."

Up to now, the government's dealings with the Black Market had been a fiercely guarded secret although Swain suspected that most of Congress was aware. But not Jamison. She had purposely been left out of the loop. The desire was for the government agencies to continue their affiliation with the Black Market without Jamison's knowledge even once she was president. This would ensure their relationship—that of the government and the Black Market for quite some time. Eight years anyway. By then, the next president would be unable to find the line between the two.

"We only want this one outcountry hospital. That's all," Cyrus Kadar said innocently. "We are not interested in being out so far. This would be just an interim step for us. Our goal of course is to be in the cities providing healthcare openly."

"What about The U.S. Government System's program?"

"Swain, you've been earning a tidy income living on the fence. The time is coming where you will have to choose. The U.S. Government Healthcare Distribution System or the Black Market. We have been patient with you. But we have our limits."

Swain felt the corner of his eye twitch ever so slightly. A tic that only occurred when the wheels of one of his plans were coming off the cart. Had the government allowed too much leeway? Given the Black Market too much freedom? Would his interests be served better by the U.S. Government if he broke his ties to the Black Market?

"Why don't you let me connect directly with your agent out there at this St. Luke's? Surely you have at least one mole out there?"

"Of course." Swain made a quick decision to agree now and figure out what to do later. "I will get you her name and computer address. Perhaps she can be of help to you."

"Don't worry about the tab. I'll take care of that," Cyrus Kadar said as they got up to leave. "And remember, you have a choice to make."

Swain headed directly back to his office. Time for crisis management.

# CHAPTER 28

As soon as Swain returned to his office he emailed the information he had promised Cyrus Kadar. Marilyn was a pretty tough cookie. Cyrus Kadar would have a difficult time getting anything past her.

Then he placed a call to Hartman. "We need to have a conversation. In person. Yes, I would say it is urgent, and it does concern your lovely wife."

Swain knew he had to find a way to protect the senator—his continued employment in the government depended on it. He needed to talk to Hartman before anything else happened.

Before he could collect his thoughts, the phone rang again.

"Swain. This is Jamison."

"Debra, how nice to hear from you. How are you feeling?"

"Actually, Swain I'm feeling very healthy and strong. As a matter of fact, I've received very good care out here. As you knew I would."

"I'm glad to hear that." Swain rubbed his twitching eye. Eye drops! He rummaged through his desk drawer for them while he spoke to Jamison.

"I have to admit this place really surprised me. And I want to thank you for directing me here."

"Oh, really?"

"Definitely. They have all sorts of interesting resources here, both medical and otherwise."

"I'm glad you are happy, Senator."

"I'm not happy," she snapped. "I didn't say I was happy. I said I am feeling well. I've learned some very disturbing news while out here. Funny, I guess you thought my being out here would mean I would hear nothing of the latest news of Washington."

"Oh?" Swain said cautiously as he switched to the remote receiver on his phone so he could use the eye drops.

"Yes, very interesting stuff. Like your slimy connection with the Black Market. And you know I have certain goals I want to achieve should I become president of this great country of ours. Well, while I've been out here I've developed some new ones."

"Very interesting, Senator. I'd like to hear about them, but I am expecting an appointment. Is there anything specific I can help you with right now?"

"Actually, there is. You can stop talking to Cyrus Kadar and his Black Market cronies for starters. And halt the impending destruction of St. Luke's while you are at it."

Silence.

"Swain, are you there? Did you catch what I had to say? I know what you and Hartman, my beloved husband, think of me." She paused. "I may have some physical problems, but they haven't affected my brain as yet. And as long as I have all my mental faculties, I will work for what I think is good for this nation."

"Senator, calm down, just calm down. I know you are feeling cut off being out there. But you'll soon be back here in Washington with Todd and all your friends who support you." Swain used the most reasonable tone he could muster.

The door to Swain's office opened. "I have to go now; my appointment is here. We'll talk again soon, I'm sure." Swain punched the off button on his phone and then looked up at Hartman as he entered the room.

Hartman appeared agitated, "We have a problem."

"Oh, yes, we do," Swain agreed, "We certainly do. What's your problem—you go first Hartman."

"My wife! She is still out there at the hospital. You can't have the government troops go in there until she is out. I'm counting on you."

"Todd, have I ever let you down? You know I haven't. So trust me, will you? Just trust me. I'm not going to let anything happen to her."

"Good. When can I see her? It's been three months. I miss her, and I need to see her."

"Very soon." Swain tried to appear thoughtful. "In fact, I'm going to send someone over tonight to get her out of there. Nothing to worry about. I have things under my complete control."

"You do?" a tentative Hartman responded.

"Of course! That's what they pay me for." Swain faked a carefree attitude.

"How are you going to handle that Cyrus Kadar fellow?"

"Who?"

"The Black Market," Hartman responded impatiently.

"I don't know what you are talking about."

"It won't work."

"What won't work?" Swain faked innocence.

"Pretending like you don't know or that my information is bad. It's bad enough we have the Underground competing with the U.S. Government's Healthcare service. Now you want to let the Black Market in? I think you've lost control and your mind all at once."

"Oh, don't you worry about me," Swain returned angrily. "The Black Market—they aren't so different from you and me. They have power, lots of it. We want power, lots of it. If the Black Market can be the one to give it to me, I'm not going to say no. I'll willingly accept and so will you and so will your wife, whether you two will admit it right now or not. Why not let the Black Market have St. Luke's?"

"With Debra there?"

"No! Of course, we'll get Debra out. In fact, we'll let everyone who wants to leave go. That will be OK. I'm sure there are plenty more patients willing to come in. Then the Black Market will owe us." Swain said triumphantly.

"Will what?" Hartman groaned. "They don't owe anyone. Don't you know that? And they don't pay their debts if they don't feel like it. And you know what, Swain? Most of the time, they don't feel like it. Oh man! I can't believe you got us embroiled in all of this. You actually think The U.S. Government will stand for this?"

Hartman sat down and thought for a minute.

Finally, decisively, he stood up. "I want out. Totally out. I want no more to do with you or any of your friends. I want totally out of this. And I want none of this to touch my wife. Understood?"

"Perfectly," Swain responded calmly. Hartman stomped out of the room slamming the door behind him. Swain looked at the door and said, "Once you're in, you're in."

The coffee smelled great. And it was wonderful to be out of the hospital and sitting in an office even if it wasn't her office. It was McClaren's. Paul sat at McClaren's desk opposite Debra. They quietly sipped their coffee considering one another.

Paul opened with, "I didn't think people in Congress had any guts."

"I didn't think journalists were ever honest."

They both laughed quietly.

"Guess we're even," Paul said quietly.

"I guess so." Debra looked up from her coffee at him, "You need me," she said.

"We need you," Paul agreed and took another sip of coffee.

"You need me to stop this mess. To stop the destruction of St. Luke's and other private, ethical deliverers of healthcare."

"That is true, but sometimes I wonder, can it ever be stopped? I mean what can be done to stop this insane struggle for healthcare?"

"You mean you don't have a plan?"

"No, actually," Paul admitted, "I don't. All this time I have been helping with communication, and I've wondered what do I want? How should healthcare in the U.S. change? I don't know. Still can't answer that."

"Amazing! All of this time you've never known what you wanted."

Debra gestured to the door, "What about him," meaning McClaren who was in the sanctuary. "What does he want?"

Paul looked thoughtfully in the direction she indicated and then back to her, "Dunno." Then he said, "I guess he just wants to be able to do things the way he wants to, without government interference."

"That's it, of course," Debra nodded. "What," she continued, "if I told you I've come around to your way of thinking on this?"

Paul just stared, thinking. Debra waited. Finally Paul began, "Well, I'd be very surprised, first of all. Then I'd wonder about your sincerity, quite honestly." He paused. "Since you've always wanted the government to take over, I would wonder how this change had come about."

"Of course, I can understand your hesitance to believe me. Yes, I did think that The U.S. Government Distribution System would work for most people. But I realize now that I was wrong. Not everyone wants to be taken care of that way."

They both were silent for a while. Thinking.

Paul spoke first, "So how do we get your friends in Washington to change things?"

"Well, first we do have to develop in writing what we want. Then I need to go back and begin circulating our 'wish list' so to speak.

Then we figure out when to vote on it and how to make it become part of U.S. Law. And we need a body."

"What do you mean? A dead body?"

"Well, not exactly. Doesn't have to be," Debra was thinking out loud. "We need a person, an unhappy person, deeply unhappy with the government system, someone who wants a change. A person who knows next to nothing about medicine. An average citizen. But someone who passionately wants alternative healthcare to be legal. Do you know anyone like that?"

"Well, sure I do, but, well, it goes back a long ways."

"No, we need someone who has suffered at the hands of the Black Market or the U.S. Government recently."

"There is a police officer's son here. Maybe that would be the way to go."

"Yes," Debra said thoughtfully, "Yes, Aaron, yes, I know him. Sounds like a very real possibility," Debra said smiling as she took another sip of coffee.

After a tearful family reunion in Aaron's room, Rufuos and Stacey had offered themselves to the staff at St. Luke's to help. Rufe was soon helping with the moving preparations. Stacey worked in records backing up the computer information. Her girls were with Aaron. Karyn had fallen asleep next to Aaron while Donna alternated between playing video games and exploring her new surroundings.

Cyrus Kadar inserted his cipher disk into his personal computer. Nobody had access to his machine just as no one ever knew fully what he had on his mind. He smiled. A smile filled only with condescension and derision. What fools most people were. As he waited for his self designed program to boot up, he gazed at his reflection in the computer screen. He knew he had a handsome face. He used his appearance to his advantage. The posture, the dress, all designed to make people think he was just another pretty face. They didn't know, couldn't see beneath his carefully designed exterior. Brilliance needs to be kept hidden. No one would possibly have expected him to reach the heights that he had.

He started as a lowly tech. Look at him now. He gazed once again at his steel gray eyes. He kept them hidden behind mirrored sunglasses most of the time. But of course, it didn't matter because no one could possibly know of his intentions.

It had all been so easy. Swain, Hartman, all the rest so interested in keeping a government run health system. Hadn't they studied economics? Didn't prohibition teach them anything? Of course, medicine had been such an emotional topic. The decision makers were totally unable to think objectively. Their constituents cried to them. Manipulated them really. So now the government controlled the dispersal of medical care. But what a lousy job they did. The doctors, nurses, techs, all too soft. Didn't use their brains when it came to the business of medicine. Where did they get the idea it was any different from any other business? They had a product. Limited resources, limited supplies. Only natural a black market would be born. At first by doctors who thought they could make money and still maintain standards. Of course they found out soon enough that wasn't so. That's when he had made his move. Climbed the corporate ladder. The corporation being the Black Market. A business like any other. We provide a service—a product. Put it in short supply, and just like any other product, the price goes up. It's so simple, so clear and so easy. Of course, everybody, including the caregivers, was hungry. Hungry for a chance to make some real money. They may think they are better than he, but they shared a common motivation. Money. And it didn't take long to make that the primary interest for the doctors who were disgusted with the pay the government gave them.

All just sitting there, waiting for an entrepreneur such as himself. Someone with a vision, an eye to the future. Just like any company, the Black Market stood ready to make a leap in growth. Up until now, they had had no permanent sites. Unlike the Underground. Now that was a group to be concerned about as a nemesis far more problematic than the government. Soon the U.S. Government System Hospitals would fold. Their financial problems were severe. And bound to get worse, what with the likes of Hartman lobbying for more money and benefits for the caregivers and then also asking for more coverage for the patients. Didn't they understand the resources were finite? Only so much medicine, equipment and brain power. Which accounted for the Black Market's continued success. A businessman knew to charge whatever the market would bear. And, of course, people being the saps they were, would spend anything for a loved one.

Cyrus Kadar looked at the paper Swain had given him with Marilyn's email address. He shook his head in disgust, crumpled the paper in his fist as he would the smallest of insects. He punched in the coded email address she had given him long ago. Not only was

Marilyn a talented doctor, she, unlike Swain, had been smart enough to see the future. Hopefully she would be at her computer. Sure enough.

He typed: The time is here. The U.S. Government plans total destruction of the site. This is wasteful as, up until now, the government has given us permission to take the site. But we want the equipment and meds as well. This is where you come in. We need you to allow our agents entry secretly into the church so we can overwhelm.

The answer came quickly: I'll be waiting for you. We will use the entrance we talked about before, Paul typed in response.

# CHAPTER 29

It had been an absolutely fine day, Debra thought, as she lay down to sleep that night. She and Paul had a plan. She knew Todd would go for it once he understood how things really were. She missed him terribly, but it wouldn't be long before …

Suddenly, she heard movement behind the curtain surrounding her bed. Instinctively she grabbed her blankets to her chest in surprise, then relaxed when she saw it was Gail.

"What is it?" Jamison asked.

"It's time." Gail answered ominously.

"What do you mean?" Jamison asked.

"I've come to get you out of here."

"But I'm not leaving. Not until everyone else does."

"I'm sorry, Debra. But I'm going to have to insist." She looked over in the darkened room at Debra's open suitcase. "Good, you've started to pack. Finish up quickly, and then we'll go. I have a car waiting."

"Gail, I don't know what you're talking about. I'm staying right here with the others. I thought you were, too."

Gail sighed, "I wanted to, but that's all changed now. I have a chance for advancement. And this is all going to be destroyed anyhow. Plus, it isn't the Government that's coming. It's the Black Market. I don't think you want to be here when that happens. They won't care that you are a senator." She remembered Swain's carefully scripted instructions. "So you see, the rest of the country needs you. Alive." She paused. "We've talked enough. It's time for us to get out of here. We don't have a lot of time."

"You go, Gail. Tell your superiors that I had already left before you got here. Just go."

"I don't think you understand what this means for me and my career. And frankly, Debra, your career future doesn't look so good. I know you have been scheming with Paul. You know how the public feels about the press. So get up and finish this packing, so we can go."

Gail watched as Debra looked over at her suitcase and then back at Gail defiantly.

"OK, if you insist." Gail reached into her purse and pulled out a gun. "I mean business, Debra. Now get up."

Debra slowly acquiesced. She went over to her suitcase and put a few more things in before closing it and latching it. She looked back at Gail.

"OK. I'll go with you."

Gail quietly backed out of the room and waited for Debra to lead. They made it without notice up the stairs, through the sanctuary and out to the parking lot and Gail's car. St. Luke's was eerily quiet. Gail told Debra to get into the driver's seat. She quickly popped the trunk to double check. Earlier she had loaded it with the medicines Swain had requested she take now. He would be pleased. She breathed a sigh of relief and slid into the passenger seat. Soon, at her direction, they were heading down the highway toward Washington, D.C.

Even though it was three o'clock in the morning, Swain lay awake in his bed. The phone rang and he answered immediately. A voice said, "The mission has been completed. We have the stock."

"What about the woman?"

"She left as planned just before we entered."

"You're sure?"

"Absolutely. She was with the agent just as you said. All went according to plan."

"Good work." Swain hung up the phone and dialed Hartman.

"She's out."

Without asking who, Hartman replied, "Oh God! Thanks Swain."

"Don't use my name." Swain hissed and hung up abruptly.

Rev. McClaren tossed restlessly. Some day he would sleep again. How long had it been since he really slept? He couldn't remember a restful night. The phone ringing was almost a relief. He answered it quickly.

"Hello, McClaren here."

"Hello Reverend. It's me, Debra Jamison."

"What could be on your mind at this time of night?"

"Actually, I'm not at St. Luke's. I'm on a cell phone out on the highway. I need you to get everyone out. Now."

"At this hour?" McClaren cried.

"Immediately," Debra said with a heavy voice. "Get everyone out. Gail dragged me out of there which can only mean they're planning the takeover very soon."

McClaren jumped out of bed. Holding the phone against his shoulder with his chin he said, "I'm already on it."

"Good. How will I find you?"

"I'll find you."

"Good, just write me at Capitol Hill." Debra's voice was calm. "And Reverend, I won't forget what you have done for me. I won't forget."

"OK," McClaren replied. But could he believe?

Swain did his best work at night. The whole world slept while he made sweeping changes. The average person had no idea what went on in the world anyway. But working at night made things much easier. Important people answered their phones. No secretaries or assistants to take up your time asking inane questions. He accomplished so much and so efficiently. There would be time for sleep later. But for now, he needed to direct. By sunrise St. Luke's and its inhabitants would be no more. The president left it to him. Didn't he always? Swain had no desire to be in politics. He delighted in his own power. He didn't need a fan club. Once the media figured out what happened in outcountry, all the most knowledgeable figures would be gone.

Yes, Debra Jamison could prove problematic. But she could be useful as well. He would wait and see. Gail would be bringing her directly to him.

"The sky always goes on forever at this hour." Debra looked over at Gail, sitting uncomfortably now with her hands tied behind her back.

"I really don't want to talk about it." Gail replied. "I'm busy drafting my letter to Congress about you in my head."

"Really? How's it going?"

"Just fine. You will be able to read the contents before an investigative committee. Soon as we get back."

Debra looked at Gail. Shaking her head she said, "You are naive. No one will be hearing your complaints. Even if you were able to take me back. Swain doesn't care about you. In fact, I wouldn't be surprised if you returned to a pink slip."

"I don't have to listen to you."

"No. You don't. I plan to go back of my own accord. Government is my life. And I miss my husband even knowing his faults," she said more to herself. Then she turned to Gail, "You could be of help to me. But you're under the control of your superiors. People who care nothing about you. They don't care if you have a job tomorrow or not. Nor do they care what happens to you if you should need hospitalization."

"How can you say that after all the government has done for you?"

"Aw, come on Gail. If I were just anybody, they wouldn't have cared a whit. But since I could be useful to them, they decided they wanted me to live. I have no illusions. They will discard me as soon as I serve them no purpose."

Gail lowered her eyes. Debra decided to be quiet for a bit. Poor girl, she thought as she looked at Gail. It had been so easy to overpower Gail. People always underestimated me, Debra thought. Swain, even her husband, Todd, whom she adored, they all thought they could control her.

Debra's cell phone rang.

"Are you safe?"

"Yes, I believe I have things under control. Should we return to St. Luke's?" Debra glanced over at Gail.

"No, not a good idea. It's going to get very hot here. Can you hang on to Gail for a while? Just till we have a chance to relocate. We may decide to just let her return."

"No problem." Debra looked over to see Gail's eyebrows raised in questioning. "We've been having a nice chat."

Gail frowned at her.

Debra just smiled sweetly. "Be careful, Paul."

"Don't worry about us. We're going to get out of this. Then we're going to need you."

Paul hung up and smiled to himself. He wouldn't want to be Gail just now. Other issues called. He headed down to the hospital

He found Rufuos sleeping next to Aaron. He shook Rufuos' shoulder gently. Rufuos awoke with a start.

"We're ready to move."

"I know," Rufuos looked over at a now very awake Aaron. "You know I have to go help these folks."

"I know Daddy. You help people. I'll be fine." He looked up at Paul.

Paul smiled, "Hi, Aaron."

"Hi, Mr. Paul."

Rufuos leaned over Aaron and gave him a hug. Then he turned to Paul, "What can I do for you?"

Paul glanced over at Aaron who was watching the men intently. With a nod of his head, he indicated that they needed to move away. They headed up the stairs to the sanctuary.

"I've received some information. It seems The U.S. Government Healthcare System and the Black Market are fighting over St. Luke's. So, we are trying to get everyone out tonight. Not the way we planned it. But our information is pretty good that the government tanks will be arriving tonight, and the agents for the Black Market will try to stop them in an effort to steal as much equipment as possible and keep them from physically destroying St. Luke's Hospital. They want it for themselves it seems." Paul shook his head in wonder. "What an irony. If I believed all the stuff McClaren believes—the Black Market here in a church or The U.S. Government—either way doesn't seem like they belong here." He paused, "Anyway, I need you to get some people together to hold these guys off until we can get out. Do you think you can do that?"

Rufuos hesitated, "I don't know."

"Maybe this will help. Follow me." Paul led him into the sanctuary and up the steps to the pulpit where McClaren stood each Sunday no matter how many made it to the service. McClaren was already there, kneeling. On impulse, Rufuos stepped back to give him privacy while he prayed. Paul kept going though and indicated Rufuos should follow. As he came closer, Rufuos realized McClaren wasn't praying. He was kneeling over a hole in the floor. The wooden lid was propped up against the pulpit, and Rufuos looked down into the hole in the floor to see a surprisingly large array of guns. McClaren looked up. "Maybe this will help?"

Rufuos nodded, "It certainly will."

# CHAPTER 30

Swain's position grew more precarious with each passing minute. He found deceit and subterfuge scintillating but only when he knew he would eventually prevail. This time he knew he had to win and win big for the government. Or they would replace him. He could not allow this. He had to fight and win. Cyrus Kadar and his Black Market organization had mushroomed out of control in part because he, Swain, had helped them grow. Cyrus Kadar, megalomaniac that he was, could not be content with the organization as it stood. Swain saw that now.

The answer, as usual, intertwined strategy and force. St. Luke's served as the perfect backdrop. The site would be attributed to the Black Market rather than to a bunch of altruistic healthcare providers, and the government's success could be plastered all over the news web pages. He, Swain, would continue as he had always done. Ever the victor.

Bolstered by the fact that they actually had weapons, Rufuos sprang into action calling Marcie, Macklin, and Matt together. They huddled in McClaren's office.

Rufuos spoke first. "We have a clear objective here. And that is to safely evacuate patients first, and second, take as much equipment and medicines that remain as possible. We need a group of armed guards to provide protection while this occurs. That's why we have called you together. Any of you by chance ever fire a gun?" Marcie pulled her jacket aside to reveal her holstered pistol. Rufuos nodded silently and looked at the other two. No response from them. He looked back at Marcie, "Well, better than nothing, I guess. OK, Marcie I want you to show the others how to use a gun. McClaren, it turns out, has weapons stored in the sanctuary, so we will use those.

They are simple to use. And it doesn't take a genius to shoot a gun. Just make sure of what you're shooting first. Marcie will show you."

McClaren appeared at the door holding a shotgun. "I'd like to help."

"What's going on, Mommy?" Aaron asked plaintively. Stacey sat down on the bed next to him and took him in her arms. She had been asleep on a makeshift cot with her daughters, but awakened feeling uneasy and had decided to check on Aaron. She knew Rufuos had been with him earlier. She had the girls with her and they jumped onto the bed to be near their brother.

"What is Daddy doing, Mommy?" This now from Karyn.

"Well, he is going to help protect everyone here including us." Sensing the seriousness of the moment, Karyn began to cry.

"Now Karyn, don't worry. It's going to be OK." Stacey rubbed Karyn's curly topped head affectionately and kissed her forehead. "We're all going to be together and be safe. Very soon," she added with emphasis. "Daddy is taking care of us, so you needn't be fussing like this. He wouldn't want us to be doing that, now would he?" She looked at each child individually. "Here, Aaron, you tell the girls a story, OK? I want to go help the others. Now Karyn, stop your crying. Look at Donna. She's not crying." Karyn glanced at her younger sister but grabbed onto her mother's shirt anyway. "Oh well," she put her arms around Karyn and said to Aaron. "I'm going to take Karyn back with me. She can watch me pack up the patients. You can read Donna a story. Maybe she'll fall asleep." Aaron put his arms around his baby sister and nodded wisely to his mother.

Back in McClaren's office now, Paul said to McClaren, "You know, Reverend, those trucks that are coming might come in very handy."

McClaren looked up from the gun he was examining, "Well, I think you're quite right about that, of course. How could we work that out?" He looked around at the others.

Rufuos responded first, "I think we can come up with something. It sure would be nice to have those trucks."

Swain knew that the Black Market would be a fierce competitor. He knew his own personal health was at risk if he went against Cyrus Kadar, but he also knew that once he was no longer useful to Cyrus

Kadar, he would be expendable anyway. Hadn't the government always treated him right? It had been especially good benefiting from both organizations, but that was over now. And the government would make sure it ultimately won. Yes, if he wanted to survive, he would have to help the government. With twits like Gail working for them, they needed all the help they could get.

Gail, that was it! Why hadn't he thought of her before? She could get word to the Underground. Let them know the Black Market was coming. That they had to help the government. They had to be made to see that the Black Market was much worse than the government when it came to delivering healthcare. They couldn't possibly want that. He opened his phone and dialed her cell phone.

The two women traveled in silence. Debra had always enjoyed driving and even though this was Gail's tiny and not very energetic vehicle, they were moving at a good clip down the highway in the direction of Washington, D.C. Just the thought of returning to her job had raised Debra's spirits. She smiled as she thought of seeing her friends. She even looked good. (She caught a glimpse of herself in the rearview mirror.) A telephone ringing interrupted her daydreams. She looked over at Gail sitting quietly next to her, hands still tied.

"Shall I answer it?" The phone in Gail's messenger bag rang insistently. She wiggled to remind Debra her hands were still tied. Debra looked at her, checked her rearview mirror and pulled the car swiftly over to the shoulder of the road to a smooth though rapid stop. With a quick look at Gail, she calmly reached for the phone, pushed the enter button and the speaker button.

"Gail is that you?" a male voice said. "Is it safe to talk?"

Debra nodded meaningfully, "Yes," Gail responded her eyes never leaving Debra's.

"Well, we have a situation. One that I think you could help me with."

Swain wanted her help? That was hard to believe.

"Go ahead."

"Are we secure here? It sounds like I'm on speaker."

"Oh, we're quite safe," Gail said cynically.

"This may be a surprise to you. The Black Market wants to take over St. Luke's."

Gail almost laughed, "Yes, I have heard that."

How did she know this already? Swain became a bit more nervous.

"Well, we can't let that happen," Swain used his most persuasive voice.

"Really? I thought that's just what you wanted."

"No, no, I don't, no, we have to get those folks at St. Luke's to understand. We can't allow the Black Market in. It wouldn't be good for anyone if that happened." Swain paused to allow this information to sink in.

"Wait a minute. Are you telling me you want their help? After you had me help you steal from them, now you want their help?" She looked at Debra for sympathy and support. Debra raised her eyebrows as if to say, now you see.

"Things change. You know that, Gail," Swain held his temper in check. "I like my job," Swain accentuated "my" clearly indicating he would take Gail down with him.

"OK, so you don't want the Black Market to have it," she answered wearily. "Does the government want it?"

"Well, not really. It still has to go; otherwise, the Black Market will find a way to get it. I want you to go to McClaren," Swain went on, "Tell him you want to deal."

"OK, and just what is the deal?"

"The deal is that we will allow them time to get out, even aid them in their evacuation. But we want their help in repelling the Black Market forces."

"How can they do that? They are doctors and nurses."

"Oh, I have a feeling that they are very capable. I'll send some government agents to help. We'll supply arms and ammo and most important, I can get information."

"OK, hold on just a second." Gail waited for Debra to press the hold button before she spoke. "What do you think?"

"I think we're heading back to St. Luke's. Sounds serious. Can't figure out if it's a trap to end us all though."

"Me neither," Gail said. She couldn't believe this. Her life wasn't supposed to be like this. She worked for the federal government. She pledged an oath of loyalty and now look at her. Tied up by another federal employee, both of them about to go in with the likes of Swain who supposedly worked for the government, but really worked for himself, Gail thought disgustedly. Debra turned the phone back on, "How much time do we have?" Gail asked quietly.

"I need an answer now."

Gail felt heat rise from somewhere inside her. Her cheeks felt warm with anger. Her voice carried the irritation to Swain, "Well, I can't do that. I'm on the highway. I will head back and talk to them at St. Luke's." Gail noticed the surprise on Debra's face. She realized her voice sounded different than usual. Sterner, harder. "Meanwhile, you start getting that help you're saying you can access."

Debra reached over and untied Gail's hands. Debra nodded silently in agreement, started the car and made a quick U turn back to outcountry.

# CHAPTER 31

"They want us to what?" Paul was incredulous.

"You heard me right," Gail responded. "They want your help in destroying St. Luke's so the Black Market can't have it."

"They are asking for your help, and they are willing to give their help to protect everyone as we leave," Debra interjected.

Paul looked from one woman to the next and back again. They were gathered in McClaren's office at St. Luke's.

"Debra, you think this is a good idea, don't you?"

"I do," Debra responded quietly. "It's a good beginning."

"Always the politician," he responded.

"I'll take that as a compliment. Yes, that's what I do." She looked at him hard. "It will give us a leg up when we finally get through this mess and go back to Washington. We—I mean—your organization," she continued deferentially, "will have helped the government. It will give you a voice. This is an opening for the Underground to come to the table later and exert pressure on the government medical establishment. I think you should take it."

Paul looked from one woman to the other and, exasperated, walked out.

He found McClaren and the others where he had left them in the sanctuary.

"I have some news for you and the others." Everything stopped, and all eyes turned toward Paul.

"There's been a new development. The government has communicated with us through Gail. Apparently her supervisor called her on her cell phone while she and Debra were on the highway. They want our help." He felt a collective drawing in of breath. "I know it seems weird. But there must be some kind of power grab between the Black

Market and The U.S. Government Healthcare Distribution System. So they need us, and in their clumsy way are admitting it. Here's the thing. They want to help us evacuate. And they want our help in repelling the Black Market forces and destroying," he turned and looked meaningfully at McClaren, "St. Luke's."

McClaren yelled uncharacteristically, "NO!"

Marcie stood up from where she had been on the floor checking the mechanisms of the guns they were planning to use and silently put a hand on McClaren's shoulder.

"It may be the thing for us to do," she said quietly.

McClaren dropped his head in defeat. "This church has been my dream. I know all of you think I'm silly." There was a collective muttering of no's from the others. "But I had such hopes for this place. I am proud of what we have done here."

"We all are, McClaren," Marcie said.

"And we can do it all again." Dr. Chambers said emphatically. "It's just going to have to be somewhere else."

"I don't know." McClaren shook his head from side to side. "I don't know if I have the energy to do it all again. I may regret agreeing to this." He looked up and made eye contact with everyone one at a time. "We may all regret this."

Paul hung back and let McClaren have his say though it didn't change anything. And Paul knew that. The others did too; he was sure.

Finally he offered, "If it's any consolation to you, Debra Jamison thinks this is a good thing for the Underground. She is looking ahead, Reverend. And maybe you should too. She says the government may listen a bit more to us; we may have more of a voice on the national level, you know, in Congress once we get ourselves settled somewhere else. We may be allowed to testify before Congress. She has already said she has plans for some changes. Some freedoms to practice medicine the way we want to."

Suddenly the whole sanctuary shook.

"We're under attack!" John yelled as they all dropped to the ground.

"Get under a pew," Marcie yelled. "It's started already."

From his window on the second floor, Rufuos saw the trucks suddenly appear. How had they come in with no lights or sound? He had been studying the horizon with his binoculars for hours. But darkness had arrived, and he had begun to think today wouldn't be the day.

More crashes and yelling from downstairs ensued. People were yelling. Then he saw them. A line of hyper speed tanks were assaulting the building. Just as suddenly, it all stopped.

John slid out from under the wooden bench dragging his gun. It felt cold and foreign in his hand. He looked at it and gripped it tighter.

"I'm going to check the back door." He stayed low as he headed to the door to the hospital. Just as he opened the door, he felt a presence behind him.

"I'm with you." Marcie said quietly.

Using the cover of fire, a group of men stealthily entered the building through the basement entrance. So quiet that even the air didn't move. Each with his own task, the men swarmed through the supply chests that had been so neatly packed quietly depleting the soon to be moved hospital of any medicines that were left, syringes and the like.

John and Marcie arrived at the basement exit only to find the door hanging open.

"They're either here or have left already," John said in a whisper.

He turned and looked down the darkened hallway.

"The meds." He said with no expression.

They heard the rustling at the same time. Marcie touched his shoulder and indicated the open door. They stepped outside and to the side and waited.

Soon they heard stumbling and hushed voices. The glow of a flashlight on the ground outside the door. John had no time to think. Should he fire? What should he do? The sound of the intruders came closer. Marcie indicated the butt of her gun. She stood behind John, but now tried to move around him, but he held his free arm up and kept her behind him. He waited. Then he saw first a foot and then the rest of a body dressed in black. He did not hesitate. He hit the first thief on the top of his head. Marcie reached around and pulled the victim of John's assault to her. The darkness worked in John's favor as he was able to get another in the same fashion. All was quiet. Then, ever so slowly, the barrel of a gun inched out of the doorway pointed in the direction of John and Marcie. John saw it first and grabbed it pulling hard bringing this next intruder out and off of his feet. The gun went off but as it pointed in the air, hit no one. Marcie reached around John and the stranger as they struggled and hit the villain on the back of his neck. They waited and listened. No more.

From her place behind the wheel, Sis Leland heard the order in her headset to stop the assault. Sis couldn't believe her bad luck. She had been in the Maryland Reserve for years, but had never pulled such a nasty and confusing duty. Now they were being told to actually help an Underground organization. Here's hoping she didn't have to look at Rufuos and eat her words.

Her commander had issued the orders not to shoot at the hospital or its inhabitants. Orders were that they were actually to protect the patients and healthcare workers as they left. Apparently, since they were willing to go quietly, the government had decided to help them and to keep the Black Market out. She knew that was the main objective. But she knew that would only help temporarily. The Black Market was growing rapidly. No one could really control it. They had too much money.

It was just at that moment that Rufuos, panning from one tank to the next, laid his eyes on Sis. He shook his head in disbelief. "You've got to be kidding. What the hell is she doing here?" he said aloud though no one would hear him. "Now what are they doing?" he muttered as he noticed that the whole operation was stalled.

Paul tapped him on the shoulder. "They're stopping!"

"I can see that," Rufuos responded not taking his eyes off the tanks.

"There's been a change." Paul said quietly as he gazed out the window.

"Really? It must be a humdinger," Rufuos responded as he continued intently visually scanning the scene outside.

"They are sending trucks to help us evacuate."

"What caused that change of heart?"

"Well, seems they would rather help us than have the Black Market take over," Paul answered.

Rufuos continued to study Sis' face when suddenly the view within his binoculars turned to smoke, and he heard Paul yelling, "They're already here." Paul went running from room to room of the second floor to where the rest of those with guns were already stationed.

"Begin firing, but over the tanks to the trees beyond. The tanks are being assaulted from the rear."

After giving orders, he returned to Rufuos who sat on the floor, back to the wall muttering over and over, "She was my partner."

Paul shook him. "Rufuos, Rufuos, you OK?!" he yelled. "We need you!"

As if from a trance, Rufuos looked up into Paul's eyes. "How can this be happening?"

"Who knows?" Paul answered. "It just is. It's happening, and we've got to stop it. I've called the government operative who is our contact. He's sending air support. Meanwhile we have to protect those tanks." Suddenly with renewed resolve, Rufuos grabbed his rifle and checking carefully through the scope began methodically firing into the trees beyond the tanks.

# CHAPTER 32

Marilyn had been holed up in her room ever since Paul became aware of her connection to the government. She didn't fear for her life, certainly. She didn't believe this group was capable of violence of any sort. She was a bit worried that they might leave her, and the government in its zeal might blow up the place with her in it. As long as the St. Luke's organization was here, she figured she was pretty safe. She knew Paul was good at getting information. And the government was sloppy in its computer security. So for the time being, she was safe. She prided herself on her medical abilities and believed in the work she did. The Underground was kept under control by the government whether they realized it or not. Through moles such as herself, the government had a good idea of the Underground and the level of care it offered which was why they had sent Senator Jamison to this particular facility. The government had an image to keep up which was why the Underground organizations had to keep moving. The government had stumbled onto a way, thanks to the McClarens and Chambers of the world, to provide national healthcare for the average American and superior service for members of Congress and other important figures.

Shook by the reverberations of the first attack, Marilyn crawled from under the bed to the window of her room and carefully looked out. Paul entered carrying a laptop which he quickly hooked up and booted up.

"What are you doing?" she asked him quietly.

"Just sending another email to your pal, Cyrus Kadar."

"He won't believe you are me." Paul didn't respond.

He typed: *What are you doing? You said you would get me out of here first.* No response came. He tried again:

*The patients are still here. Your forces are attacking. That wasn't supposed to happen. If I get out of here safely, is there a place where we can meet?*

Still no answer. Paul slammed the laptop shut. "Well, so much for your friend."

"He's not my friend," Marilyn looked over at Paul.

"Sure, sure," Paul answered. He picked up his laptop and had his hand on the doorknob to exit when they both looked up as they heard the jets fly in. The noise of the low flying jets was deafening. They both ran to the window. The tops of the trees were lighting up with twinkling flashes!

"They must be seeing a target!" Paul said.

Marilyn did not respond. She walked over to her bed, sat down, and wondered what she would be doing if she ever got out of this mess safely.


"I wouldn't go out there just yet," McClaren warned. He stepped in front of Rufuos as he headed for the exit. They had all reconvened after the air assault on the Black Market forces.

"I have to," Rufuos said. "I have to check on my partner. She was driving one of the trucks." McClaren nodded, understanding, and he stepped aside to allow Rufuos to pass.

"So senseless," McClaren said to no one in particular as his gaze followed Rufuos outside.



Paul found Matt, Marcie, Chambers and Macklin on the roof. John, while looking through binoculars, motioned Paul to come over. He took the binoculars from him and saw what John already had spotted. Four guerilla type figures were making their way around the government tanks to the woods beyond using the government tanks for cover. Paul handed the glasses back to John.

"We got three of them already. We can take them," John said.

"Aren't you a surprise!" Paul said.

Marcie said, "I'll go with John. We'll follow them."

"I know you both are anxious to get out there, but let's just let them go. It's not worth losing you two. I guess those jets didn't get all of the Black Market operatives," Paul said, and then, "Where is Rufuos?"

"He's gone outside," John said. "Checking on his partner, who coincidentally happened to be in one of the trucks that was supposed to help us evacuate."

Paul sighed, "OK. You know what to do, right? We're to provide cover for the U.S. vehicles as the Black Market forces are going to try to destroy them first."

"Don't worry; we will stop them," John said. He looked at the others, "We can do it. Right?"

"You aren't afraid," Marcie said to John.

"No." And strangely he wasn't.

Paul regarded John for a moment. And then, "OK, go ahead. Get in position. I'm going to check downstairs and make sure the patients are safe."

"I've never shot at anyone before. Only at a range. How about you?" Marcie said after Paul had left.

"You are ahead of me. I never even held a gun before!" He ran his fingers over the barrel of the gun. "And I never even hit another person let alone use the butt of a gun."

"What are you doing here?"

"What do you mean?"

"I mean you were all safe and secure. Working at the Wellness Center. Nice place to live. Pretty wife."

John didn't take his eyes off the clearing between the trees and the entrance to St. Luke's.

He shrugged. "I guess I can't explain it. I just know that this is a better place for me. I only know that what the Underground does helps a lot of people, and the Black Market has to be stopped."

"But your home?"

"This is my home now. I've chosen it as much as it chose me. And it's not about money."

"Oh, I get it. By that you mean that's all it is to me? You don't know me."

She stopped talking and focused on the area below.

There was silence for a bit, but then, "I've never really been tough like you," he said.

"I'm not so tough," she said softly. "I've always just had to pretend." Their eyes met. She looked down and said, "It would be nice if I didn't have to, anymore." She smiled briefly and turned to look back through her binoculars.

"Shhhh!" she said. She carefully placed the binoculars between them. She nodded to him as she peered over the edge of the roof and saw a group approaching. This was not as Paul had predicted. These men appeared heavily armed. She took one last look at John. He at her. And they commenced firing.

Rufuos heard the shots and hit the dirt next to Sis' truck.

He crawled up to the side away from the shooting and searched frantically for a sign of life.

"I'm here!" said an angry voice followed by a hacking cough.

"Sis!" he said, so relieved. "Are you hit?"

"No! They shot out my engine though. And I couldn't figure out what was going on. How about you?"

"I'm fine, just fine. How did you end up here anyway?"

"I'm in the reserves, remember?"

"Yeah, well you sure had me going there for a bit. I saw the smoke in your truck."

"I'll be OK. Nothing a few days at the spa won't fix," she said.

"Come on, let's get out of here."

The day dawned with the hope that comes at the end of an endless night. It had been too long. John and Marcie sat in the dirt next to four dead strangers who had planned to destroy them and anyone else who kept them from taking St. Luke's. Why they had cared so much John couldn't explain. Even so, he felt miserable. He had been sick after seeing their cold white faces. He knew he needed to get control of himself. But he just couldn't right now. Later. Later, he would find the right corner of his mind in which to place this particular horror. And he would find the strength to go on. St. Luke's now belonged to him. He turned to look at Marcie. She had been quiet. He thought she looked quite innocent.

"What?" She turned to look directly at him.

"Nothing."

"C'mon, you're staring."

"Just thinking."

"OK, so?"

"You aren't so tough."

"What do you mean by that?"

"Hey now, don't go off on me."

"I'm not going off." She started to stand up, but he firmly pulled her down next to him.

"I'm not afraid of you."

"What's that supposed to mean." Fire in her eyes.

"He gently touched her face and than pulled his hand away before she could say anything.

"You're not so tough."

Marcie put her face in her hands and cried.

John put his arm around her and they sat quietly among the ashes and dust.

People were starting to come outside to survey the damage. St. Luke's still stood. There were bullet holes all over its white facade. No one had really slept. The doctors had gone inside to prepare the patients finally for the move to the next facility. Some slept wherever they could find a cot. But most just listlessly wandered around. Too much had happened to allow sleep.

Paul found McClaren kneeling in the sanctuary praying. He sat down in the first pew and waited. Soon McClaren joined him.

"We were strong, weren't we?" McClaren said.

"Steadfast," Paul replied. "The government is sending more trucks and people to get us out of here. They've found us a place. A place of our own. So you can build up a new St. Luke's. I'm sorry though. For security you'll have to pick a new name."

"That's OK by me. I think I have a name all picked out," replied McClaren.

Cyrus Kadar arrived at his bank as soon as it opened and made a sizable withdrawal of funds. Aruba was nice this time of year. He needed a vacation.

"Hello Aaron," Gail said. She nodded to the rest of the family including his parents. She looked at Rufuos, "Could I talk to your son for a minute?"

"Sure." Rufuos stood and went over to stand next to Stacey and his girls.

Gail went over and sat next to Aaron. "How are you this morning?"

"I'm fine." Aaron said in an uncharacteristically soft voice. "Don't feel like telling any jokes though."

Gail smiled, "I'm sure not. That's OK, Aaron. I've brought someone to meet you. Do you know who this is?"

He looked at Jamison who now came closer to join them.

"No," he answered.

"Don't be afraid. We're here to ask you for your help. This is Senator Jamison." Gail accentuated Senator.

His mouth formed an o.

Gail smiled, "That's right. She is very important. She works in the Congress. You know about that, don't you?"

"Yes, we learned about it in school."

"Right, and you know that in Congress they try to make this a better country, right?"

"Yes, they make bills."

"That's right," Senator Jamison said. "Good for you! Now guess what? We want to take you to see the Congress, if your mom and dad let us, that is. We want you to tell them all about your stay at St. Luke's. How you have gotten better—everything—would you be willing to do this?"

Aaron looked over at his dad who smiled reassuringly. "Can my dad come?" he looked from Gail to Debra.

Debra smiled, "Of course, bring the whole family."

# EPILOGUE

The Honorable Debra Jamison reporting to a joint session of the U.S. Congress:

Senators and Representatives:

Thank you for allowing me to speak to you today. I believe you will find what I have to say startling as well as important. Its importance cannot be undermined. For what I have to say will affect all of us and the generations of Americans to come.

Some of you may be aware that I have been suffering from a major illness over the last five years. Perhaps you are wondering if I have tabled my plans to run for president. Happily, I come before you to assure you that my health improves daily (*applause*). I am happy to report that I believe I have received in the last few months the best medical care in the world (*more applause*). I see my colleagues from the health reform subcommittee smiling quite satisfied smiles. I hasten to inform you that the fine care I received was not at the hands of the U.S. government (*silence*). Where did I go to receive this care, you are wondering.

www.ingramcontent.com/pod-product-compliance
Lightning Source LLC
Chambersburg PA
CBHW050523260626
47157CB00004B/1447